A Diagnosis
for Two

Published by Marian Steel LLC
P. O. Box 286
Harrison, ID 83833
www.lavarsteelart.com

Printed in the United States of America
First Printing, 2021

ISBN 978-0-578-87507-1

Library of Congress Control Number: 2021904974

Acknowledgment

We owe a great debt of gratitude to those who offered assistance in editing this book—Julie Jones, Jolene Wallace, and John Gray. Each has a unique view of dementia and screened our writing through that sieve. It is another example of how difficult things in life can be accomplished with the help of others. It's true in caregiving as well as in publishing a book.

Dedication

For those who care deeply and
give selflessly . . . caregivers.

Table of Contents

A Diagnosis for Two

Why?

It may seem odd to begin a book with this question. However, most adults need to know why they should care about something before they learn new information. Likely, your "why" is related to experiencing the heroic task of supporting, advocating, and caring for someone with dementia— most commonly Alzheimer's disease. In this challenge, you are not alone since it is estimated 5.8 million Americans have Alzheimer's dementia, and it is projected that nearly a million new cases will be identified yearly.

Making the risk factors more personally relevant, at age 45 women have a 1 in 5 (20%) lifetime risk of developing dementia, and men have a 1 in 10 (10%) lifetime risk. With Alzheimer's dementia, subtle symptoms develop years-even decades-prior to diagnosis, so even more cases are in the process of developing. Also the number of dementia cases is expected to rise dramatically because individuals are living longer with various chronic conditions that lead to dementia. Even aging is a risk factor. We are all at risk for developing this disease. Hopefully, understanding how prevalent dementia is and will continue to be, you have generated your own "why."

As a physician, why do I care? Weekly . . . sometimes daily . . . I have to address the issue of dementia. I'm on the front lines of diagnosing a difficult, life-changing disease. Although the patient maybe disturbed by the findings, I have so much compassion for the caregiver who will carry an incredible responsibility. Witnessing the caregiver's tears, I want to help. However, the minutes available to doctors and patients in an office visit don't allow for the extended coaching that I would like to offer.

Collaborating on this book is my attempt to reach out to patients and caregivers in order to answer their questions that they haven't even formed yet. Each case of dementia, whatever the cause, is unique. Likewise, your questions and concerns will be different than others. Caring—one human to another—is my "why" for contributing.

As a caregiving survivor, why do I care? Everywhere I encounter individuals who are struggling with the same fears, frustration, and fatigue that I experienced. If my understanding can help others, then I'm willing to share strategies that helped me not only survive but also find joy in the work of caregiving. It has been difficult to write about myself in the context of these challenges. However, being transparent and letting you see this role through my eyes is the only way that I know how to help you personally since we can't sit down together and chat. No magical approach makes caregiving easy although there are ways to manage it. Offering help to those who struggle as I did is my "why."

The contents of this book are the result of a collaboration between Jared Helms, DO and Marian Steel, PhD. Anticipating the situations that you and your loved one will likely encounter, the authors offer suggestions from their own experiences with and perspectives of dementia. This book is not a comprehensive treatment plan for the patient nor a script for the caregiver. Rather, it is guidance for addressing difficult situations and encouragement for caregivers as they fulfill a demanding role. It is help for two—from two.

A Diagnosis for Two

Introducing the Physician

Jared Helms, DO

My career in medicine began in 2002 as a student at the Des Moines University School of Osteopathic Medicine. This program appealed to me because of the holistic philosophy of osteopathic medicine. Specifically, the body is a unit; no part functions independently. The body has an inherent capacity to heal itself and maintain its health if the right conditions exist. Promoting wellness is Plan A; whereas, treating disease is Plan B. Like most physicians, I was idealistic, optimistic, and hopeful that I could help people "be better."

After graduating in 2006, I began an internal medicine internship and residency. Daily, I saw patients who were in the early stages of chronic illnesses. Seeing the initial expression of disease and understanding the predisposition for advancement, I tried to coach patients. My intent was to help them understand their conditions so that they could help themselves by making lifestyle changes. Unfortunately, many patients' health declined as they continued to make poor choices and instead, relied upon prescription drugs and supplements for health.

In my internal medicine practice, I find many similarities. At follow-up appointments for chronic health problems, I inquire about what a patient is doing for high blood pressure, diabetes, etc. I'm always astonished when I get the response, "I'm taking my medication every day." I remind the patient that prescribing medication is my contribution. The patient's part is to make necessary lifestyle modifications that will support improved health. Clearly, many want medication rather than education. Although medical advancements occur regularly, the fundamental principles of wellness are in the control of individuals.

My interest in preventing illness and disease has increased as I practice medicine. I want my patients to live longer without the impairments of chronic illnesses, which often advance into some type of dementia. Some patients have the misconception that a predisposition for a disease is a destiny. When discussing a diagnosis about diseases such as diabetes, cancer, or dementia, a common response is, "I do not want that." Others offer a reluctant acceptance of an inevitable fate citing a family history, injury, or other extenuating circumstance that destined them to a particular diagnosis. When making a diagnosis of dementia, these types of reactions are disheartening. If a fatalistic attitude delays a diagnosis and the dementia becomes well established, a tragic outcome is unavoidable. Then the only option is disease management.

A diagnosis of dementia affects more than the patient. It is a diagnosis for the spouse, the family, many friends, and caregivers. I understand personally because I witnessed the decline and death of a loved one who suffered with Alzheimer's dementia. I not only feel compassion for the patients and their families but also empathy. Accordingly, I would love to sit with each of them and offer comfort and advice as needed. Unfortunately, the time is not available in an office visit. The next best thing that I can offer is to share some recommendations in this book.

Hopefully, you will find the information useful in changing your view of this disease and adopting new ways of approaching the day-to-day struggles of living with this condition. Repeatedly, I will stress the importance of seeking an early diagnosis because the greatest benefits are found in early identification and intervention.

A Diagnosis for Two

The Diagnosis

Some confusion may arise when using terms for various types of dementia. To clarify, "dementia" is a generic, umbrella term for several neurodegenerative conditions. Since the most prevalent type of dementia is Alzheimer's disease, the terms "dementia" and "Alzheimer's" are often used interchangeably. A definitive diagnosis of Alzheimer's dementia requires a brain biopsy that reveals neurofibrillary tangles and beta amyloid plaques, so this type of brain disease is usually diagnosed clinically. As part of the work-up for Alzheimer's dementia, other types are considered and then ruled out. Sometimes pre-existing conditions may lead to a different diagnosis initially, such as Parkinson's dementia, which is an expected progression of Parkinson's disease. Recurrent stroke or repeated transient ischemic attacks (TIA) would make a vascular dementia much more likely initially. Differentiating among the various types of dementia may be useful in order to optimize treatments and reduce risks of unnecessary medications. However, in early disease — in the mild cognitive impairment stage — there are common pathways stemming from lifestyle choices that lead to a dementia syndrome. Thus, the terms dementia, Alzheimer's, and Alzheimer's dementia are used interchangeably.

Warning Signs

Every day in my internal medicine practice, patients and their families pose common questions and express concerns. When does "dementia," "forgetfulness," or "cognitive decline" really start? Is it an expected, normal part of aging or an inevitable expression of genetics? Can the changes be reversed? Some memory concerns are brought up nonchalantly as part of a follow up for chronic diseases such as diabetes, hypertension, heart disease, kidney disease, etc. Sometimes it is subtle. "Dad forgot to take the garbage out last week. He thought that it was the next day." Other times it's alarming. For example, family members had been waiting for their father to meet them in Utah, but he never arrived. The next day, they received a call from a motel manager informing them that their father had arrived at a motel in Eastern Idaho the night before. Upon trying to check out, he did not know where he was nor where he was going. I have learned that if someone brings up the issue at any level, there is already a problem. Some type of degenerative process has begun.

Cognitive impairment is the progressive loss of function in at least one of the following major categories: memory, language, visual-spatial function, behavior, or higher level executive function. Because symptoms can be vague, it is common for a spouse or adult child to recognize a loss in one of these areas and accompany the patient to an appointment to express concern about their observations. The patient may not be as acutely aware of the deficit because he or she has learned to adapt to the gradual loss of these functions and essentially "cover" it well.

Many people worry about becoming forgetful because the tendency is to think of dementia as purely a memory-loss problem. However, it is much more complex. Forgetfulness can be a normal part of aging, and several things can make anyone forgetful regardless of age. In residency when we talked about identifying early dementia, we often said, "If they remember that they do not remember, there is probably another condition mimicking dementia." Everyone has episodes of walking into a room and forgetting what was needed. Most often that is due to distraction—losing track of the present because too many things are running through the mind. It's normal if that happens occasionally. Dragging a loved one to a doctor with every episode of forgetfulness could create relationship stress. However, a daily occurrence of similar memory lapses are less likely to be normal, and the goal is to notice and address these conditions early.

Look for a change in learning new skills or recalling recent events. One of the hallmarks of Alzheimer's dementia is clear recollection of distant memories whereas new memories are more difficult to retrieve. Consider the brain as a field of tall grass. As you walk through the grass, a trail develops. Walking the path repeatedly, you crush the vegetation that eventually does not regrow, and the trail becomes permanent and easily followed (old memories). If you walk a new path once and forget to go that way again, then the grass quickly stands up and fills in with no evidence it was ever disturbed (new memory).

Observe changes in routines or behaviors. Was a simple, repetitive task routinely done but now is neglected? Are there changes in sleep, activities, or paying bills? It is more likely that there is something else causing these changes, so it is worth a conversation. You may uncover some underlying anxiety, depression, developing sleep issues or some other disorder. If not, it may be one more reason to seek a medical consultation. Further, we know that these underlying conditions can contribute to the development of cognitive impairment.

Situational stressors such as a retirement, death of a spouse or friend may lead to confusion and forgetfulness. These effects usually fade with time, but if they persist, it is time to seek assistance. Other more obvious signs include the following: becoming lost in familiar places, asking the same question or repeating the same story, becoming disoriented about time, people, or places, or neglecting personal safety or hygiene.

In medicine we talk about activities of daily living (ADLs) and instrumental activities of daily living (IADLs). ADLs are considered the basic necessities to care for yourself within your own home. The instrumental activities of daily living require more complex thinking and organizational skills. I often see family members begin helping with IADLs feeling that their loved one just cannot keep up physically, but there is often a cognitive problem that is being overlooked or minimized. I include a breakdown of these activities because it will help you track the continuum of disease progression. The following are the typical ADLs and IADLs. As a family member or friend, you are more likely to recognize a loved one's difficulties in these areas. Particularly, be aware of the activities as they relate to the stages on the FAST Scale. (See next page).

Activities of Daily Living (ADL)
Basic Necessities of Self-care

Walking	Getting around the home or outside—"ambulating"
Feeding	Getting food from plate into the mouth
Dressing & Grooming	Selecting clothes, putting them on, and managing personal appearance
Toileting	Getting to and from the toilet, using it appropriately, and cleaning oneself
Bathing	Washing face and body in the bath or shower
Transferring	Moving from one position to another-from bed to chair, standing up from bed or chair

Instrumental Activities of Daily Living (IADL)

More Complex Thinking and Organizational Skills

Managing Finances	Paying Bills and Managing Finances
Managing Transportation	Driving or arranging other means of transportation
Shopping	Shopping for clothing and other items
Meal Preparation	Performing all tasks required to prepare and serve a meal
Housecleaning	Cleaning kitchen after eating Keeping living space reasonably clean and tidy
Home Maintenance	Keeping up with home maintenance
Managing Communication	Telephone Mail
Managing Medications	Obtaining medications Taking as directed

In assessing the progression of Alzheimer's or other types of dementia, the FAST (Functional Staging Assessment Test) scale is used, which in part references these ADLs and IADLs.

Stages		FAST Scale
Stage 1	No Difficulty	Risk factors for developing hypertension, diabetes, heart disease, history of stroke, tobacco use
Stage 2	Forgetting location of objects	Subjective work difficulties
Stage 3	Decreased job functioning	Co-workers notice difficulty Difficulty in traveling to new locations
Stage 4	Decreased ability to perform complex tasks	Examples: planning dinner for guests, handling personal finances
Stage 5	Requires assistance in choosing proper clothing	

Stages		Fast Scale Continued
Stage 6	Decreased ability to dress, bathe, and toilet properly	a: Difficulty putting clothing on properly
		b: Unable to bathe properly; may develop fear of bathing
		c: Inability to handle mechanics of toileting (i.e., forgets to flush, does not wipe properly)
		d: Urinary incontinence
		e: Fecal incontinence
Stage 7	Loss of locomotion, consciousness, and speech	a: Ability to speak limited (1 to 5 words a day)
		b: All intelligible vocabulary lost
		c: Non-ambulatory
		d: Unable to sit up independently
		e: Unable to smile
		f: Unable to hold head up

As family member or friend, what stage would concern you? The majority of patients brought in for evaluation are already at Stage 5 or 6, closer to the end than the beginning of the scale. Now the family wants to "address the issue before it becomes a problem." It's disappointing to hear family members comment that they saw something years before but didn't think anything of it or dismissed the changes as part of normal aging.

Addressing Concerns

Family members or close friends are the ones most likely to recognize a departure in a loved one's functioning. When you see signs that concern you, don't be timid about addressing the issue. It's unlikely that a medical professional will identify early indications of brain dysfunction in a short office visit. Cognitive assessments are not part of routine follow-up appointments for hypertension, diabetes, sleep apnea, or heart disease. An abundance of simple cognitive tests can be done—even at home, but an extensive evaluation is much more complex. Insist on dementia testing because no comprehensive examination is done by a physician without someone raising a concern to warrant the assessment.

Several years ago, Medicare implemented the "annual wellness visit" designed to provide preventative-care screenings. As part of that office visit, a patient

receives a simple cognitive evaluation. Although
the specific test is not mandated, some interpret the
regulation as "complete" if the patient can identify the
correct day of the week/ month/ year and repeat his
or her address. If there are difficulty with those items,
then clearly, we have missed opportunities to identify
a problem and treat early. Another simple assessment
is composed of drawing time on a clock, and recalling
a list of three items. Although possibly useful in
identifying that there is a memory iue of some type,
it is neither sufficient for a diagnosis nor a basis for
dementia treatment.

Since the Medicare wellness screenings don't generally
start until age 65, it is not reasonable to rely on
identifying dementia early through this means. When
you have cause for concern, schedule a doctor's
appointment specifically for a cognitive evaluation so
that the physician has enough time to consider the
complex issues that may mimic deficits and begin the
necessary testing.

The Diagnostic Process

My approach is to identify reversible causes of
symptoms by evaluating multiple aspects of the
patient's health. An initial evaluation includes a review
of the patient's medical history and a critical look
at lifestyle. We discuss possible depression, poor

sleep, physical inactivity, alcohol, tobacco, and other substances, including some prescription medications known to contribute to dementia. An evaluation generally consists of a more detailed cognitive test, a physical exam, and blood and urine tests. Although there are no blood tests that definitively diagnose dementias, the review and work-up are needed to rule out reversible causes of dementia. The tests may identify other issues that can present as dementia syndromes, such as B12 deficiencies, thyroid conditions, diabetes, etc. The chance of reversing the cognitive impairment from any cause is better when these problems are addressed as soon as possible.

Brain imaging such as a CT scan or an MRI of the brain are also part of the work-up. The imaging may reveal microvascular disease or atrophy (shrinking) of the brain. These are often referenced by the radiologist as "age-appropriate" or "expected" findings for age. The sad truth is that these are not normal. They are the results of decades of disease. It might be a common finding, but a diseased brain should be considered neither "appropriate" nor "expected."

Brain imaging is still a developing area of medicine. For example, it has been proposed that the amyloid plaques, which are the hallmark of Alzheimer's dementia, are not necessarily the cause of the disease but rather the body's attempts to protect fragile brain cells against harmful lifestyle conditions. The other issue to keep in mind with imaging is that we are looking for structural problems, anatomy. We are neither looking at the physiology nor the function of the brain. Although it's possible to do a functional MRI, they are listed as investigational and not part of the standard of care nor usually covered by insurance. Ultimately, a functional MRI does not change the treatment offered to the patient.

Although family members typically accompany a spouse or parent into the exam room, any distractions can interfere with the assessment. For example, when a patient cannot answer a question on the cognitive test, a loved one may try to "help" by supplying cues. It's important to remember whose memory is being assessed. Only participate by contributing information if the doctor requests your input.

Understandably, when adult children take their parents to the doctor's office for cognitive testing, the parents are often defensive. In these situations, it is useful for the family to provide written accounts of incidents or observations of the family's concerns and then allow the parent to come into the exam room alone.

When I ask patients about the activities of daily living, universally, they respond that they are able to do all of those things. For example, they claim to "cook dinner" but usually do not reveal that cooking dinner means going to Burger King or pulling out a pre-prepared meal from the refrigerator. When a family member is present for the evaluation, some bickering can occur when trying to correct the information supplied by the patient. A written log allows the family's concerns to be addressed in a clear, accurate, and respectful manner.

Treatment Options

The common belief regarding dementia is that there is no cure. Dementia syndromes are considered chronic disorders and therefore, regarded as progressive diseases. The accepted view is that once dementia is well-established, it is likely too late for treatment to have a meaningful effect. Although some studies show promise in dementia treatments from a pharmacologic standpoint, the current medication options are only temporary measures that can neither stop nor reverse the disease. Treatment is considered successful if it slows the rate of decline–but decline is still expected as part of the normal course. However, the medication may slow the dementia long enough so that the patient will die of a heart attack, stroke, or other event and avoid needing a care facility. This paints a very bleak picture of dementia syndromes — an inevitable decline. A reality that is disheartening to family members and physicians alike.

Some seek relief in well marketed, over-the-counter supplements. Many of them are marketed with the claim to be "clinically proven" in treating dementia. If treatment were as simple as taking a pill, the numbers of newly diagnosed cases of dementia wouldn't be as high as it is. I am not opposed to my patients trying the supplements. Perhaps an individual has a nutritional deficiency (which should be identified during the initial testing) that can be corrected with these supplements. The placebo effect is very real. Sometimes it is just a sense of relief that they are doing something to treat their condition. When my patients ask about these products, I have them read the ingredient list. Then I ask if they would be able to get the same nutrients through food. Ultimately, the final claim for the supplement is always, "This product is not intended to diagnose, treat, cure, nor prevent any disease."

The truth about dementia and many other health problems is that they can be prevented. Prevention is the cure. I often hear patients remark, "I had a parent with Alzheimer's disease, so I will probably get it." However, the environment and lifestyle choices can enhance or retard the expression of those genes; a genetic predisposition for dementia is neither an inevitable fate nor a predictable aspect of aging. Lifestyle changes in diet and exercise hold the greatest promise for preventing and even reversing dementia. This approach protects bodily systems even before an actual disease has developed.

Identifying a reversible cause in lifestyle, learned behaviors, or habits can be helpful. Any damage inflicted by poor choices is not necessarily permanent since the body is continually regenerating cells and tissues. However, some tissues regenerate at a slower rate, so improvement may not be recognized immediately. Degeneration is a process and so is regrowth. As the understanding of dementing disorders increases, it's clear that prompt intervention is better every time.

The first consideration is diet. It is well-established that a whole-food, plant-based diet rich in antioxidants supports brain and vascular health. The MIND diet (Mediterranean-DASH Intervention for Neurodegenerative Delay) and Mediterranean diet are rich in antioxidants and provide the nutrients that the brain needs without having to take a supplement.

Stay active. Have you ever been told that osteoarthritis particularly in hips and knees is a risk factor for heart disease? Probably not, but we know that a sedentary lifestyle is a major vascular risk factor. Physical activity not only increases blood flow to the brain but also increases a protein called brain-derived neurotrophic factor. This is not as complex as it sounds–neuro refers to neurons or the basic cells of the brain. Trophic means to grow. BDNF is a protein that is generated by the brain that stimulates nerves to grow. More growth means more connections and an active brain. Less growth means dementia. How much do you need? A brisk walk of 30 minutes at least 5 days a week is enough to increase blood flow and change the very structure of the brain.

Dementia paints a bleak picture and is not an easy conversation. Since the typical demented mind will show subclinical signs years before diagnosis. Physicians are already treating conditions that contribute to dementia for decades before diagnosis. For example, diabetes, hypertension, high cholesterol, heart disease, kidney disease, sleep apnea are considered pre-dementia conditions. Recognizing these conditions as precursors, perhaps there would be a bigger push to reverse the disease. Yes, I said reverse.

Once a treatment plan is initiated, everyone is eager to see improvement. It can be discouraging to attempt major lifestyle changes and feel as though there is no immediate payoff. Your loved one may strongly object to changes in lifestyle and medications. It is necessary to create a balance between quality of life and the conflicts of imposing unwanted changes. The degradation took years to build up; the solution will take years to reverse.

Whether you want it or not, chances are that you will be affected by this condition. Where are you on the spectrum? Predementia? Recently diagnosed?

A Diagnosis for Two

A caregiver facing a future of increasing demands and isolation? When should you be concerned? Simply put — NOW. Be concerned NOW. Prevention is the CURE.

Recommendations for Caregivers

As a physician, I see many patients with dementia, and a caregiver usually accompanies them to an office visit. The signs of fatigue and stress are often apparent in the caregiver. The wellbeing of the caregiver is vital to offering another person care, a heroic task. Since crucial aspects of health are easily neglected, it's worth a reminder of the principles.

First, your diet is the fuel that you're giving your body to do heroic work. Because I always recommend a plant-based Mediterranean or MIND diet for your loved one, I urge you to follow that eating plan as well. It leads to lower levels of systemic inflammation, lower instances of depression, and increased physical and mental resilience.

Exercise is an easily-neglected element of wellness. Make time to be active during the day; just being busy with your many duties will not suffice. If you and your loved one could take a walk daily, it would be incredibly beneficial to both of you. Otherwise, find an activity that you like and MAKE time to do it every day.

Don't neglect yourself emotionally. Take the time to pause and reflect on things that are personally meaningful to you every day through meditation, journaling, reading, or prayer. It's a way to center yourself so that you don't lose track of what matters most. Some activities may overlap so that you are actually doing two things at once. For example, some may go for a walk and engage in prayer or meditation while moving.

Give some thought and consideration to these lifestyle suggestions because they will not only improve your health during waking hours but also improve your sleep quality. Restorative sleep is essential. Sound sleep begins with being able to rest safely without concerns that disrupt slumber. Sometimes the caregiving role becomes an issue during the nighttime because of wanderings and episodes of your loved one's fitful sleep or agitation. If you wake exhausted and unrefreshed, then your new day is lost already. Recognizing poor-quality sleep is a cue to make needed changes and is an issue to discuss with your physician.

At a doctor's appointment, be open and realistic about your feelings. It is easy to minimize some of your own needs and say that you're doing fine, but if you are overwhelmed and not sure how you are going to get through the week, talk about it. Spiraling into depression will negatively affect your sleep, diet, and activity patterns, and consequently, both you and your loved one will suffer. Additionally, don't ignore your own health concerns. If you have chronic diseases that need treatment, make arrangements to get help so that you can take care of your own medical needs. You have to be mindful of your own physical and mental health. Finding family or friends to help you by spending time with the patient will provide the respite that you need to take care of yourself.

It can be difficult to stay connected socially when friends and family are reluctant to visit and engage a loved one who isn't able to interact as he or she once did. The lack of social contact creates isolation for the caregivers of dementia patients and is probably harder on them than it is on the patient and is detrimental to both. As the caregiver, invite friends and family to visit and offer suggestions of ways to include the patient in conversations and have an uplifting, cheerful interaction. Through these efforts, you may be able to create a social support system that will be available to you in a crisis. Even when you're doing everything right, challenges will arise, and having supportive family and friends can make an amazing difference.

Caregivers often ask for suggestions about creating an environment that will provide the greatest comfort for a loved one. The most important element to consider is creating a calm and pleasant environment. Without meaning to cause distress, caregivers can add to confusion and agitation by trying to "straighten out" a loved one. Consider how much you like being told that you are wrong. Imagine that your brain is not working correctly, and no matter how much you are told you are wrong, you cannot understand why or how to fix it. That is a very tense feeling and can rapidly escalate situations. Unless there is a safety issue, there does not have to be a "right or wrong."

Another potential point of conflict is in viewing dementia patients' hurtful comments or distressing behaviors as being driven by malice. Quite often I hear a caregiving spouse recounting a hurtful behavior as though it had been done on purpose. It's not difficult to imagine the hard feelings that accompany that belief. I have seen many divorces in older couples that stem from these types of situations. As a physician, I suggest that they reframe situations. This requires the caregiver to keep the disease in perspective by first, recognizing the effects of dementia and second, not taking incidents personally. If you as a caregiver can maintain a more positive focus, your anger, frustration, and resentment will be much easier to manage. Since you are the one whose brain is functioning normally, it's up to you to manage situations for the best outcomes.

Visualizing elderly patients with or without dementia in facilities, you can easily picture residents in various states of alertness seated on furniture and in wheelchairs and watching television reruns of the *Golden Girls* or *The Price is Right*. I can imagine neither myself nor one of my loved ones enjoying that activity nor benefiting from it. As a physician, I have worked with skilled nursing and assisted living facilities and know that they try to implement activities for the residents. Although they try to individualize the sessions, it is difficult given the regulations and limitations of the facilities and staff. Therefore, coloring pictures, playing bingo, and tossing a beach ball become ways to pass the time.

As caregivers and families search for ways to help a loved one with dementia, my first recommendation is to look to the individual. Start by reminiscing— talking about the past and activities that they enjoyed. Maybe you will uncover something exciting for the patient that you can implement with a little creativity. Going through old pictures or treasure chests may lead to discussions of fond times and could even be useful for creating physical or digital scrapbooks with stories that could be passed along to grandchildren. This adds purpose and meaning to activities and can be mentally stimulating.

Think about how you can incorporate previous hobbies and activities with current physical limitations.

A Diagnosis for Two

Perhaps a loved one has been an avid golfer but can walk only a few feet now. Using foam golf balls and a short putter, you could create an indoor course that is navigable in a wheelchair. Technology offers the options of video games and virtual golf experiences, which could allow a patient to participate in this favorite activity with neither the physical demands nor the coordination of a full swing.

Using a personal example, I enjoy skiing. I participated occasionally in my youth, but it was accompanying my daughter on her fifth-grade ski trip that brought me back to the slopes. Returning to the mountain now, I reconnect with that memory even when I'm alone. Over the years, I have developed many other mental and emotional attachments to skiing that go well beyond the physical experience. Skiing will be part of my life as long as I am physically able. If the time should come that I need a walker for mobility, my children have been instructed to cut off the ends of my skis so that they can become skids on my walker. Although watching ski movies may not seem like a normal activity for the elderly, it would be more meaningful to me than watching a sitcom or game show.

We all have enjoyable activities as well as those that annoy or agitate. To help identify pleasing activities, explore and adapt favorite pastimes. Although infirmities of aging may pose barriers for participating in hobbies, some creativity on the part of caregivers or other family members can provide adaptations to make involvement possible. Perceiving individuals as having neither the energy nor capability of participating in physical activities is a form of bias. When dementia patients feel that they are becoming old and worthless, they withdraw socially to a greater extent and experience increased depression, which leads to an acceleration of dementia symptoms.

As a caregiver keep an open mind and look for opportunities to incorporate enriching activities into the daily experiences of your loved one.

A Diagnosis for Two

Considerations as Dementia Progresses

As dementia diseases progress, agitation is a common concern that I hear from caregivers. Indeed, episodes in which anger and confusion escalate can become dangerous to both the patient and caregiver. Several strategies can help you in your efforts to manage the situation. First, keep calm yourself. Do not escalate the situation by addressing anger and agitation with your own anger and agitation. Remember that this is someone you love and someone who has loved you. Look for possible underlying problems since a dementia patient may not have any other means of expressing him or herself. Consider if there is an unmet need, such as, hunger, thirst, or fatigue. Look for any signs of an infection that requires treatment. Even small amounts of common substances considered benign and "normal" to us, such as alcohol and caffeine, can trigger agitation in the cognitively impaired mind.

Rather than trying to stop behaviors and illogical thoughts, try to intercept and redirect them early. Once a situation has begun, it can be difficult to handle, so recognizing early signs and preventing an episode is the best approach. Keep a record of possible triggers for past incidents of agitation and track approaches that worked best. Using reason and logic to calm a brain that has disconnections may be futile since this part of the patient's brain may not be able to process rational thoughts.

Accessing other areas of the brain through various means can be beneficial. Music and auditory stimuli can be powerful tools. Even if patients have difficulty processing words and thoughts, music can recreate emotions and feelings. Most of us have favorite types of music and respond best to those that have pleasant associations. These pathways are well ingrained even after most of the brain's executive function is lost.

Smells can be incredibly calming as well. Think about walking into a room that has foul dog odors as opposed to walking into a home where freshly baked cookies are cooling or the fragrance of a freshly cut Christmas tree fills the air. The responses are visceral reactions; we do not have to think about them; they just happen automatically. Reactions are related to different memories and emotions that drive behavior. Why not take advantage of this response? Without scientific validation, some studies have shown that the smell of lavender reduces stress, anxiety, and potentially, even pain. With your knowledge of and experience with a loved one, you undoubtedly have many other thoughts about ways that you can soothe and distract. These ideas can become part of your tool kit for dealing with distressing situations before they escalate.

Agitation is a symptom that you should discuss with a physician because of its potential for danger. As with any condition, it's best to implement lifestyle and non-pharmacological interventions first, but underlying conditions which may be driving the agitation should be reviewed and considered. Low doses of medications which enhance serotonin in the brain are especially helpful for frequent episodes of agitation. Specifically, citalopram and trazodone are commonly used because of low side-effect profiles.

Episodes of agitation may advance into psychosis with visual or auditory hallucinations. Even if the hallucinations are not disturbing to the patient, further evaluation and disease management are necessary. Some delusions expand to the extent that the patient recognizes neither family members nor him or herself in a mirror. New episodes such as this can be distressing to both patient and caregivers and should prompt additional evaluation. Every case of dementia has its unique expression of symptoms. As a caregiver, you have to be the detective and keep track of how to manage the care of your loved one. It's a tremendous responsibility.

Someone with Alzheimer's dementia or other types of dementia may develop sundowner's syndrome, or as it is sometimes called, "late-day confusion." The exact cause of this problem is unknown, and its expressions are varied. Sundowning occurs later in the afternoon and evening and includes a number of behaviors that include anxiety, aggression, confusion, pacing, and/or wandering. Several conditions can precipitate these behaviors, but when sundowning becomes an issue, it should be brought to the attention of the patient's physician because an underlying health condition may be causing the symptoms. In my experience, this condition can be the breaking point for a solo caregiver because sleep is seriously disrupted.

Most caregivers find that they need help at some point in the disease progression. If you wait until the assistance is required immediately, it may become a great frustration. Although early stages of the disease may require only slight modifications, I recommend that as soon as you realize that you are the caregiver for a demented patient, you should devise a caregiving plan. In spite of implementing heroic, lifestyle changes and even the use of pharmaceuticals, no approach offers a guarantee that it will stop the disease progression.

Hoping that tomorrow and the next day will be better is not a practical approach. In reality today is the best day that you will likely experience. You must identify how much you are capable of doing — NOT how much you are willing to do. Almost everyone is willing to do anything possible to care for a loved one even to his or her own detriment. It's best to assess as objectively as possible how much you are physically, emotionally, and mentally capable of doing. Planning early can help you identify the point at which you may need help. This approach allows a caregiver to give advanced thought to whether that is a part-time full-time, in-home caregiver or placement in a facility. It takes time to research, identify, and locate the resources that you may need in the future.

Caregiving for another human is at least a full-time job. In early dementia stages, caregiving may not seem like a huge burden. Of course, in these early stages, your loved one is still somewhat functional with activities of daily living and perhaps even instrumental activities of daily living. For example, they are still able to drive a car, help with grocery shopping, laundry, and other household chores. As the disease progresses, there may be difficulties with having your loved one "help" with these activities. When tasks are done incorrectly it leads to frustration as you have to undo and redo the work—effectively doubling your work as a caregiver. Family and friends want to help, but the help that they can offer may not be what is needed.

With some advanced planning, it is easier to guide those who are willing to assist you.

Available community resources may be difficult to discover. Although you might expect physicians to be well informed and effective in connecting you with resources, they may not be knowledgeable about options either. It is not part of the typical medical training, and the primary role of a physician is to diagnose and treat conditions. However, speaking candidly with your doctor may reveal a need for home health services, which could provide short-term, intermittent care although it is not intended for long-term support.

Start your search with the Office on Aging. Every community or at least every state will have an agency that helps coordinate services and offers support to caregivers. You may find other support groups for caregivers of dementia patients. Though dementia is a very individual disease and a unique experience for the patient and caregiver, you are not alone. It may seem disrespectful or uncomfortable to talk about a loved one who is behaving in unusual and disturbing ways. However, support groups for caregivers can be a safe place to express your frustrations and fears. Further, it may be beneficial to hear about others' experiences and learn about approaches that they use in caregiving. You may hear something that sparks your imagination and encourages you to try a useful approach or activity that you had not considered before. These group sessions may help you to see your caregiving role from a new perspective and even help you identify safety issues for both the patient and yourself. In a group discussion, you may see that you are trying to do too much.

As a physician, I know that the caregiver is in trouble when two aspects of self-care are compromised — sleep and happiness. Although I mentioned the importance of quality sleep already, I will remind you of the key role of sleep in wellbeing. Without sleep the brain and body cannot heal, and if your brain is in a constant state of distress, then you cannot appropriately respond to situations nor process information. Fatigue and frustration breed fatigue and frustration and lead to exhaustion and resentment. If sleep is disturbed because the caregiving demands become 24/7, you are in trouble.

Similarly, if you are unhappy with the situation, then the caregiving becomes a chore that you "have to do" rather than a labor of love that you "want to do." The resulting resentment leads to poor care for the patient (as well as yourself), regret, and feelings of depression. I have seen this scenario play out to the point that when a demented patient is admitted to the hospital, a spouse says, "Enough is enough," and moves out of state.

I have also witnessed spouses as caregivers who, after agonizing about the decision, realize that the caregiving role has exceeded what they can do. With this realization he or she thoughtfully places a loved one in a carefully selected facility where he or she is cared for and safe with 24/7 care for basic needs. This decision can be extremely difficult until you apply the "safety standard." When you can no longer provide the kind of supervision and care that ensures that a patient is safe, it's a clear decision. Your first responsibility is to keep a loved one safe. Then placing a loved one in an appropriate facility that is right for both of you is not giving up—not abandoning. It is the right thing. You can still spend as much time as possible visiting with your spouse or loved one, but the total care is no longer on you. With a clear decision point of safety, it is much easier to plan for the time when additional help will be required. It also lets you communicate with clarity to other family members when you have done everything that you can do by yourself.

Some families are reluctant to consider residential care for a loved one because of the cost involved. Others feel that they have made promises never to place a loved one in a facility. Both of these issues are best addressed with early discussions and planning. I have had patients who need to be placed somewhere, and because the family has delayed any investigations and considerations of facilities, no spaces are available close by. I can't urge you strongly enough to plan for the evolving roles in caregiving for a dementia patient.

The Physician's Final Thoughts

One of the most satisfying aspects of being a physician is helping others to live their lives healthier and longer. However, the limited minutes in an office visit often don't allow for the kind of considerations that I have provided in this book. One last topic that I want to address is your ongoing caregiving role. After the death of a loved one to whom you have devoted your time and energies as a caregiver, your life may seem empty. This individual was a constant companion, your primary responsibility, and your major social contact. In one event, all of those connections become severed. Therefore, I want to offer some encouragement and reminders about your new responsibilities of moving on.

Work on revitalizing your own health. Review my recommendations on lifestyle factors that promote healthy bodies and brains. Having watched a loved one suffer with the effects of a brain-damaging disease, you will have an added incentive to protect yourself by adopting healthier lifestyle habits in all of the areas that I mentioned. Remember that prevention is the best way to deal with dementia. Watch for any worrisome signs and have the courage to address your concerns early.

Grief is a natural emotion that follows the loss of a loved one. No one is suggesting that you will feel relief rather than grief. What I am concerned about is that your grief does not become depression. Please share your concerns with your doctor if you're having difficulty coping. For some spouse caregivers, the death leaves them alone. As humans we are better if we can be around others. If you joined a support group during your caregiving role, they will still be there for you. This will also give you a place to meet new people and make friends. Your longtime friends are still available. When friends ask what they can do, think of a way for them to help you; you will both feel better. Let others into your life.

Another recommendation that I have is to find something happy or enjoyable in each day. Some who live alone get a pet for company. Caring for a pet can fill a void left by the death. This could be a good time to take up a new hobby and learn a skill. It's important for your brain to continue to learn, and new hobbies sometimes create additional social connections. Many caregivers miss the intrinsic satisfaction of making another's life better. The kindness that fills the heart when serving others is healing and can be a source of great satisfaction. You can still find ways to be of service to others. These are only suggestions of things that I have observed some of my patients doing. Be kind to others . . . and to yourself. Life is meant to be lived joyfully . . . even in hard times. As a caregiver, you have given a precious gift to another. Now you have more to offer others . . . and yourself.

A Diagnosis for Two

Introducing the Caregiver

Marian Steel, PhD

My training and professional experience is in education. I have several degrees in this field, including a PhD. However, no educational experience ever taught me quite as much as my caregiving role that ended when my husband LaVar Steel died with Alzheimer's dementia in May 2016.

I had many typical caregiving experiences, but my lack of familiarity with Alzheimer's dementia kept me from adopting and acting upon many commonly held assumptions. Learning about dementia primarily through experience, I relied heavily upon my instincts. I never viewed my husband as "gone." Even without the later breakthroughs that verified what I had sensed, I saw LaVar, the man, the individual.

Two years after LaVar's death, I published his drawings that represented his artistic expressions of Alzheimer's disease—his firsthand account of suffering with a disease that most often silences its victims. Frequent requests for "my story" followed the book's publication because LaVar was a well-known artist and a retired art professor. My refusals were based on reluctance to make a personal experience public; it was too raw — too close. Also, I didn't know how to expose my role as a caregiver without being disrespectful to LaVar. Further, I had no interest in reliving situations that filled my days and broke my heart.

Many who read the book *SEE WITH YOUR EYES – HEAR WITH YOUR HEART, LaVar Steel's Expressions of Alzheimer's Disease* asked me questions relating to their own caregiving responsibilities. Feedback about the impact of my observations and suggestions has motivated me to share some experiences in order to help others. It is in that spirit that I write. This book is not my memoir. I selected incidents so that others could see this role through my eyes and to provide context for some of the strategies that helped me in caregiving.

Possibly the most important thing that I have to offer is a perspective change, a different point of view. With memory loss, speech difficulties, and behavior peculiarities, it's understandable to assume that someone who is suffering with a dementing illness is "gone." Really . . . where would a human being go? Our dogs never seemed troubled by the changes; they didn't care that LaVar had a devastating diagnosis; they loved his company and scratches. Love for LaVar was NOT GONE.

During the last weeks of caregiving, a couple of events profoundly changed my understanding. These incidents are examples of what is known in adult education as a disorienting dilemma—an unexpected incident that enlightens someone that a current perception is inaccurate. Thus, a disorienting dilemma opens an individual to transformational learning. My former understanding of Alzheimer's disease was that someone with dementia loses awareness of people and events around him or herself. Repeatedly, I heard, "Oh, yes, my (dad, mom, sister, husband, wife, etc.) died with dementia, but he or she was gone for years before death."

The first disorienting dilemma happened on May 1, 2016, about three weeks before LaVar died. After more than a year and a half of knowing neither my name nor my role, I showed him a picture from our wedding day and asked, "Do you remember this?" First he looked closely, intently at the photo and then at me. After repeating this process a few times, he said clearly, "I know who you are." I pressed him to tell me who he thought I was. With great effort he said, "Wife." Even though I knew that LaVar struggled to use any words,

I queried, "Do you know my name?" After stammering over the "M," he said, "M . . M . . . arian." I was completely dumfounded. I assumed that this memory was completely gone along with so many others. However, this was not a momentary recollection. To the last day of his life . . . in the last moments that I shared with him . . . he called me by my name.

Another disorienting dilemma occurred four days before his death when LaVar created a caricature from a photo of himself as a young man. Not even imagining that he was capable of purposeful communication, I exclaimed, "Why did you ruin the picture?" He just pushed it toward me with a gruff, "Here." Passing by my dresser the next morning, I glanced at the photo and had a flash of insight. He had communicated his reality. He couldn't see well because of macular degeneration. Alzheimer's dementia compromised his speaking ability, and the squiggly lines represented confusion in his mind as well as his environment. This became a breakthrough, and what was for me, a Helen Keller/Anne Sullivan moment of understanding. It was shocking.

Later, holding up the picture, I told LaVar that I understood and now realized that he was communicating with me. I asked him to please keep sending messages because now I was looking for them. That same morning, he pantomimed his impending death. Each night thereafter, he drew messages in which he tried to incorporate words.

All of the months that LaVar had been drawing, he must have been deeply frustrated by my lack of understanding. After his death, I viewed the drawings with a transformed perspective. Then I understood that he was sharing his personal hell artistically and had created a first-hand account of Alzheimer's dementia through his second language—art. I didn't look for messages because no resource ever suggested that it was even possible for him to converse. Since I'm not an artist, I had no concept of how powerfully and deliberately artists communicate through visual images. Even though it's impossible to determine how much an individual with dementia remembers, I know that it's reasonable to assume that he or she is aware.

In sharing vignettes of my experiences, it's obvious that I didn't perform the role of caregiving perfectly since I didn't understand so many aspects of dementia. My best judgment was not sound in many instances. Candidly, no one can adequately prepare another for the complexities of caregiving; answers are meaningless until the questions arise. However, my own creativity is often sparked by others' solutions. It is my hope that my experiences will inspire and encourage other caregivers' vision.

A Diagnosis for Two

Signs of Change

In a time of change, the unknown and unexpected often create confusion and stress. Therefore, it's understandable to provide an explanation that is less threatening. With neither knowledge of nor experience with Alzheimer's disease or any other type of dementia, I didn't recognize slight oddities in LaVar's behavior as early signs or symptoms. It was less threatening to assume that it was some other cause that was more age related. I watched in dismay as symptoms appeared and increased.

In early 2010, LaVar mentioned that some memory lapses bothered him. However, his performance on a memory screening test was so outstanding that the doctor suggested that LaVar proudly display the results on our refrigerator door. He was relieved; I was reassured. Nothing had ever made me wonder about his cognitive abilities since he managed our finances and paid the bills. Our checking account was never out of balance, and no payments were ever delinquent. LaVar busily created in various mediums in his art studio. However, his mother had suffered with Alzheimer's dementia for at least 10 years before her death, so the possibility of dementia lurked. It was less distressing to attribute departures in normal behaviors to the typical frailties of aging. It's difficult to identify something with clarity when not looking for it.

As an aging individual, LaVar had several conditions that offered easy explanations for oddities in his behavior and functioning. One day he forgot to pick me up for a scheduled meeting. Standing outside the office building, my agitation grew as the time for the appointment approached and passed. Eventually, LaVar arrived and apologized for being late and explained his tardiness with the claim that he didn't hear the time mentioned. It was reasonable to accept his explanation since it's impossible to remember what was never heard.

Indeed, hearing loss could have explained other departures from normal routines and predictable behaviors. Although we enjoyed eating at restaurants with friends and family, LaVar became increasingly inattentive in conversations. Certainly, ambient noise interfered with the effectiveness of his hearing aids, but in retrospect he seemed to lose interest in what was going on around him. For a time, I tried to bridge the gap by repeating parts of the conversations while facing him and using exaggerated lip movements.

When something created laughter, I tapped LaVar's arm to gain his attention in order to repeat the punch line. The two of us chuckled briefly before rejoining the group chat. When he began looking away while I was trying to "translate" the conversation, the futility of my efforts became apparent.

The opportunity to eat lunch together was welcome. Routinely, LaVar drove to my office and called to let me know that he was there waiting whenever I was available. He followed this practice for years, but suddenly, he began showing up in my office. At first I was surprised, but he said that coming upstairs gave him a bit more time with me as we rode the elevator together. With such a tender sentiment, why would I question its validity? Another view of the situation emerged as LaVar stopped answering his flip phone. It wasn't a complicated "smart phone," because he only had to flip it open and say, "Hello." To ensure that he could hear the phone, I turned up the ring volume and performed trial runs by calling him while we were in the car together. Finally, I realized that using his phone had become too complicated, so he had navigated around the obstacle.

Admittedly, I was a spoiled wife. LaVar welcomed me home from work each evening with a glorious, home-cooked meal. Balancing his day with time in his art studio and the kitchen, he accomplished magnificent creations in both settings. Food was yet another medium of artistic expression. As late meal preparations became more frequent, his apologies for losing track of time seemed logical.

Travel time in our car had been especially enjoyable with interesting, stimulating conversations. When LaVar drove, I positioned myself toward him when speaking. Hearing was better in his right ear, so it seemed logical that it was easier for him to hear in this relative position. When he became a passenger more often than the driver, I noticed a decrease in the amount of conversation. It was less distressing to assume that the cause was the poor hearing in his left ear along with the fact that I couldn't direct the sound of my voice toward him as I drove. In earlier years, we both enjoyed listening to audio books, radio talk programs, and other entertainment in the car. Somehow the sounds around him became disturbing noise rather than soothing entertainment. LaVar often turned off the sound system.

As I traveled for work, LaVar often accompanied me. He typically sat outside a classroom or a conference room and read while I made a class visit or conducted business. Sometimes he walked the hallways of school buildings where adult evening classes were in session. As we drove home following site visits, LaVar shared what he had observed or read. Gradually, his activities changed. Sometimes he opted for staying in the car rather than going into facilities with me. On other occasions, he came into classrooms so that he could be near me. The dialogue of the past became more of a monologue. Again, I dismissed the change as a hearing difficulty.

A loving, protective husband, LaVar felt that his presence provided safety for me whenever I traveled. Accompanying me to out of town conferences, he usually dropped me at my meeting location, explored on his own for the day, and returned to pick me up. Then at dinner, we shared the events of our day. Increasingly, his contribution to the reports was minor although he listened intently to me. In the company of my colleagues, LaVar became quieter and rarely contributed to conversations even though everyone tried to engage him. Although he was generally a reserved man, LaVar was a generous host and an agreeable guest, so his social disconnect became awkward for everyone. I tried to offer polite explanations. Hearing loss was always an understandable excuse for his lack of participation. It even allayed my own concerns.

Later LaVar's travel routine changed. Instead of dropping me off, he suggested that I should take the car so that I wouldn't be "stranded." He insisted that he was trying to finish a book that he was reading. During lunch breaks, I often returned to check on him. Sometimes I found him in the hotel lobby, but mostly he remained in the room. On one occasion,

A Diagnosis for Two

I walked into the hotel and noticed that LaVar was seated in the lobby with his suitcase on his lap. When I approached him, he said, "The hotel told me to get out of the room." At the front desk, I was informed that LaVar had left the room abruptly when someone from housekeeping asked if he wanted the room cleaned. He took his briefcase and an empty suitcase with him. Dismissing this odd incident as a "hearing problem" wasn't reasonable. This time my uneasiness didn't subside. Other uncomfortable changes began to appear that couldn't be dismissed by hearing loss, poor vision, nor losing track of time.

A strong, resolute individual, LaVar did not let emotions overrule his reason. At first there were only glimpses of this instability. As I had some surgeries on my knees, LaVar, who was normally very capable of running the household, became rather immobilized. He didn't cook at all—a huge departure for someone who regularly made beautiful dinners. On one occasion, he abruptly left my hospital room when someone else arrived to visit. He gruffly declared that he was not needed. Looking back I recognize that LaVar was having difficulty managing his emotions. Although my recovery improved his overall functioning, sensitive situations always exposed this vulnerability. As LaVar's cognitive abilities declined, it seemed that his emotions became more pronounced and volatile.

In January 2014, we added another dog to our household—a beautiful beagle puppy named Lucy. We already had a beagle Mimi that LaVar had patiently trained into a perfect pet. Thinking that he could work his magic again, I left Lucy to the training magician. Things did not go well. Lucy was reluctant to potty train and displayed many other neurotic behaviors. LaVar stopped coming to pick me up at noon, so I came home to fix lunch and check on everything. Regularly, I came home to reports of "Lucy damage," which included chewing 11 pairs of my shoes. LaVar seemed clueless about managing this little furry nightmare. Closing our closet door didn't seem like an obvious solution until she ate the tassels off of his favorite shoes. Managing a challenging dog was too much for him.

When I realized that LaVar had stopped going out to work in his studio and sat in front of the television, I was concerned. He protested that he was tired and needed some extra rest. Often he sat on the loveseat and turned on the television after dinner. He selected a favorite show and settled in for some viewing. Sometimes he sat on the coffee table and stared intently at the screen. Soon I noticed that he stopped changing the channels. He claimed that he didn't know how to operate the remote. That seemed too far-fetched to be true.

A Diagnosis for Two

To inspire LaVar to return to his studio, I asked him to make some rattles for Christmas presents. For many years, he had created ceramic figures that made a ringing noise when shaken. Expecting that LaVar would begin working at his potter's wheel, I was surprised when he began cutting up exotic woods that he had purchased and stockpiled over the years. One day I noticed a four-foot-long piece of black walnut sticking straight out of a door. Climbing a ladder, I had to use all of my might to extricate the shaft of wood. When I asked LaVar what happened, he shrugged and nonchalantly offered, "I don't know." Alarmed, I asked, "Would you please not use power tools unless I'm here?" He said, "Nope."

Then each day as I left home to go to work, anxiety went with me. To allay my concerns, I called LaVar whenever I had a minute. At times, I returned home because he didn't answer the phone. On a couple of occasions, I found him slumped over on the couch in a sound sleep. When it was difficult to rouse him, I took him to the doctor to look for a cause of the problem. No test results identified any areas of concern, and LaVar couldn't express anything out of the ordinary. Now the disquiet that I had felt at leaving him home alone grew. Finally, I had to admit that something was wrong. My discomfort became greater than the dread of a diagnosis.

The day that LaVar took a memory test in our doctor's office remains vivid. His inability to perform simple tasks was difficult to witness; I turned my head so that LaVar didn't see the tears that dampened my purple scarf. I tried to be discrete because he did not know how to handle my emotional reactions any better than his own. Leaving the doctor's office on the day of his diagnosis, I had mixed emotions. On one hand, I felt relief at knowing why LaVar was exhibiting odd behaviors. Conversely, it was certain that the downward spiral of life would continue and eventually end with his death. No other explanation could ease the reality—it was Alzheimer's dementia—my new life's companion—'til death do us part.

When a scan showed that something was indeed happening to LaVar's brain, we opted to try medications that could potentially help to slow the progression of this devastating disease. It was only a glimmer of hope. Perhaps the placebo effect became a bit of solace for me as I looked for any sign of improved functioning. Honestly, I was dosing myself with large amounts of optimism.

In order to learn about the disease, I searched for answers in many resources. Since Alzheimer's dementia compromises communication, the ravages of the ailment were primarily documented through the perspective of the caregiver. Nothing that I read, watched, or heard suggested that LaVar's individuality was intact. Without a first-hand account of the disease, it's rather left to the imagination to explain odd behaviors and experiences of someone who is afflicted.

Television documentaries portrayed the difficulties of caregiving in graphic detail. The fear and dread created by watching exhausted individuals struggle against hopelessness shattered me. Frankly, after watching many of these programs, I found that the information created more distress and anxiety than hope and peace. I came away with the belief that Alzheimer's disease is a tragic illness; it's a diagnosis for two—one has the disease and the other suffers.

Reading about the dehumanizing effects of dementia filled me with dread as I tried to imagine losing my husband while he was still alive. None of the sources provided insights nor offered helpful suggestions for finding joy in the difficult experiences that lay ahead. Some suggested that I tell everyone that LaVar had been diagnosed with Alzheimer's dementia so that they wouldn't think that he was just crazy and mean. Other books recommended that our family and friends should be informed and organized into a caregiving team. I came to expect that Alzheimer's dementia would turn him into a disappearing human being. Nothing ever suggested that he would still be aware no matter how impaired his functioning became.

Consciously or unconsciously, the anticipation of a change keeps one looking for the signs. Since I did not recognize the signs of Alzheimer's dementia, options for potential early interventions were lost. Also, believing that nothing could be done anyway, I wasn't as proactive as I should have been. The effects of dementia increased vigorously.

A Diagnosis for Two

Experience — My Teacher

As Alzheimer's dementia impaired LaVar's ability to act independently, the reminders and oversight of earlier times transitioned to full-time caregiving. It seemed that a diagnosis should provide more predictability regarding the disease and its progression. However, I learned that every person who suffers with any type of dementia reacts differently, and decline is variable. Daily my life experience and creativity were tapped in meeting the challenges of the moment. I learned about dementia the hard way . . . from experience, life's ultimate teacher.

While I prepared to leave for work one morning, LaVar stated emphatically, "I don't want to be alone." Without enough notice to implement any other solution, he came along. This option was never one that I had considered because my focus was on maintaining stability at home while working until my early retirement date. After looking through magazines and books for a couple of days, LaVar began sleeping — snoring — on my office couch. Knowing that this passive activity was neither good for him nor an appropriate backdrop for my work, I stocked one of LaVar's briefcases with watercolor pencils and various art materials. Then I asked him to complete some drawings for a future writing project. Although he was not fond of just drawing, he purposefully began work. His deep concentration became apparent as his "working tongue" swept across his bottom lip. The wisdom that guided my approach was knowing LaVar as a creative individual who loved to be busy. Inadvertently, these materials became his means of communicating through his second language—art.

Since LaVar had been a prominent member of the College of Southern Idaho's campus community, former colleagues and friends began stopping by my office to visit with him. He seemed happy to see them and took pleasure in showing his drawings. One of his friends asked, "What were you thinking when you drew this one?" LaVar was never inclined to explain his work, but now he didn't have the verbal abilities to do so. He just returned a blank look.

Taking LaVar to work with me was an unexpected, unplanned adaptation that provided an odd respite from the chaos of daily occurrences at home and alleviated the anxiety of leaving him alone. He and

I settled into a routine of getting ready and going to work together where he busily completed numerous drawings each day. We came home to eat lunch and take care of our dogs. Fortunately, the routine worked because we enjoyed being together.

Beyond work, LaVar was never far from my side. When I went to the beauty salon, he sat nearby as I got my hair cut, colored, and styled. He went shopping with me wherever and whenever I went. During my last dental appointment before he died, LaVar sat near me and held my foot while my teeth were being cleaned. I accepted his company happily, and it eliminated his discomfort of being separated from me. Even while he was declining in every possible respect, I loved being with him because I saw Alzheimer's dementia as a malady not his identity.

When work meetings required out of town travel for several days, I had no reasonable option but to take LaVar along. Alerting the host about the situation, I was given approval to bring him. He seemed comfortable accompanying me to the meetings since he was acquainted with my colleagues. Usually, LaVar would have found a comfortable location outside the meeting room and waited patiently. On this occasion, however, he sat next to me at the conference room table, opened his briefcase, and began drawing. He selected black permanent markers and began filling sheets of paper with black swirls. Soon the room filled with fumes; we were all light headed; no one addressed air-quality concerns. None of us tried to decode his artistic communications because we assumed that he was just doodling mindlessly. In retrospect, his dark drawings quite accurately represented the meetings and expressed the tension that most certainly filled the environment as each regional director negotiated the coming year's funding. No other series of drawings ever resembled that unique set.

Because LaVar came to work with me each day, household chores were primarily done on the weekends. He loved to do laundry, but I noticed that he didn't always add detergent. The agitation that accompanied my oversight or inquiries about his process was unpleasant. Therefore, I just provided some shadow assistance, waited until LaVar left the laundry room, and then added the detergent myself. It was a departure from the normal routine, but it created no conflict and left his autonomy intact. Vacuuming was typically LaVar's household chore. While mopping and dusting, I noticed that he repeatedly vacuumed a three-foot area of carpet. Watching this oddity, I waited for him to move on. When he didn't advance, I called him away to do something else. These incidents and others alerted me that skills, once mutually beneficial, were becoming unavailable. Other unpredictable changes in LaVar's ability to function required numerous adaptations on my part. It became a time of learning many new skills.

Learning the Language of Dementia — Beyond Words

Communication is central to human interactions, so effective caregiving required learning to converse in unconventional ways. It wasn't glaringly noticeable when LaVar lost the ability to write, but his increasing frustration in speaking was painful to watch. Initially, his conversations with me were okay because we usually talked about common concerns, and I used my understanding to supply elusive words as he stammered in search of a term. Other verbal exchanges were possible if I initiated them and supported LaVar's attempts to share his thoughts. He seemed to enjoy my monologues and sometimes offered feedback or input in the form of facial expressions or occasional words. Speaking aloud gave me the sense of having discussed a problem with him and provided greater clarity through the "conversation." Previously a patient listener, LaVar received extremely high marks as a husband with Alzheimer's dementia.

LaVar's initial withdrawal from conversations in public or noisy environments became compounded now by his complete disinterest. Previously, he watched and lurked in group settings, but now he quietly focused on eating or observing other activities. My attempts to get his attention by touching his arm had no effect. He didn't even pretend to engage. Sensing his disconnect, acquaintances, friends, and even family members seemed uncomfortable, and some dodged potentially awkward situations by avoiding us. With a side glance at LaVar, some occasionally asked me, "How's he doing?" Possibly the inability to communicate is central to the tragic misconception that someone afflicted with dementia is "gone" and not aware. As LaVar's ability to use words faltered, I learned to understand his unique expressions of wants and needs through careful observations that often required repeated attempts.

I learned many related communication lessons while caregiving. One was the powerful impact of emotions transmitted through tone of voice. While preparing for travel one morning, I became annoyed about something that had nothing to do with LaVar.

Although none of my irritation was about nor directed toward him, my tone of voice expressed displeasure. When I returned from dropping our dogs at the boarding kennel, LaVar was back in bed. Coaxing him to get up only resulted in his pulling the sheets and blankets up to his chin. Failing in my efforts to get him up and dressed, I canceled the travel arrangements and waited for him to calm down. I urged him to get dressed later that day—no luck. The next morning, I enticed—definitely not. That evening I pleaded—no way! That was final. It was my fault, a communication disaster that made LaVar upset about absolutely nothing important. The only part of my words that he understood was the frustration in my tone of voice. He had no way to sort out that it wasn't about himself. It became an unforgettable reminder to monitor my emotional expressions.

Similarly, unexpected events could produce disturbing reactions. As we prepared to eat dinner at home, LaVar's awkward reach toppled a glass and sent a cascade of liquid across the tablecloth. Seeing the mess, LaVar looked distressed. Because of his reaction, I placed a hand on his forearm and offered a cheery, "Oh, dear." LaVar was calmed and helped me clean up the spill. It was challenging at first to manage that kind of self-control, but eliminating the resulting agitation made it worth the effort. Appreciating the potent effects of tone of voice was a powerful lesson that served me well as a caregiver.

A Diagnosis for Two

Although an unpleasant feature of a difficult disease, I learned that agitation was another means of communicating. Some referred to outbursts as a "mood" or a "behavior," but in observing, I realized that LaVar was communicating a need or frustration that lacked expression through other means. One day LaVar accompanied me to a haircut appointment. He was moody as I drove home and immediately removed his clothes and got into bed when we arrived. Since it was only afternoon, I asked what was wrong. He yelled fiercely, "You took so long it hurt to pee." His outburst of unpleasant and illogical behavior prompted me to look for a message. Thinking that it could be a symptom of a urinary problem, I took LaVar to the hospital where a kidney stone was discovered and treatment began. Reflecting upon other episodes of agitation in previous months, I realized that this problem had been ongoing and a likely cause of other outbursts. Although some causes of agitation defied explanation, I learned to look for an underlying problem instead of regarding the outburst as bad behavior. Learning to decode these communications provided me with valuable insights as a caregiver.

In an effort to meet his needs, I constantly looked for ways to connect with LaVar. Touch became another useful means of communication. Walking together, we touched either by linking arms or holding hands. Beyond an expression of affection, the physical contact offered some protection for him. Even without preventing a fall, I could ease his landing without injuring myself. Another benefit was that I could feel increased tension in his muscles if he became anxious or upset. With this early alert, I could intervene before a problem escalated into something more difficult to handle. Touch was like Morse code.

Beyond the information available to me through touch, I learned that touching me was comforting to LaVar. During moments of quiet relaxation at home, I stretched my legs across his lap for a leg and foot rub. He often drifted into a brief nap as his hands slid from my knees to my feet; it was a double win. Touch also came to the rescue when LaVar became anxious during car trips. Sensing his restlessness as I drove, I extended my right hand and asked him to massage it. Touch never failed to calm him—I loved it, too.

Although my touch was calming to LaVar, contact with others had a positive effect, too. LaVar and I sat in the chapel one Sunday after navigating the complexities of getting him into a suit and putting on a tie. As we waited for the service to begin, an elderly friend who also suffered with dementia walked by. The man unexpectedly reached out, took LaVar's hand in his, and said, "How are you, my friend?" LaVar didn't say anything in return, but the touch of his friend completely changed the mood. It was a beautiful expression of kindness and friendship. It exemplified the power of touch.

A Diagnosis for Two

Because Alzheimer's dementia is not a pretty illness, it should probably come with cautions: "Warning: Some images may be disturbing." "Don't stare." Beyond the cognitive effects, physical symptoms appear; facial expressions change and reflect confusion. As coordination becomes compromised, shuffling steps replace a purposeful gait. Indeed, it's possible to cover one's eyes in order to avoid witnessing the decline of another, but choosing to look away can cause social blindness. Used perceptively, eyes are a powerful means of honest communication and an invaluable source of information.

Looking into LaVar's eyes, I saw his emotions rather than a lost soul. I perceived his distress as well as the tenderness that characterized our relationship. His defiant stare signaled his unwillingness to comply and a withering glance expressed a rebuke. In moments of distress, LaVar's eyes communicated, "Help me." Observing, I had advance notice to intercept a behavior that was sure to follow. Conversely, the twinkle in his eyes was an unmistakable expression of pleasure and happiness. I saw many things that I didn't want to acknowledge, but forcing myself to look — to see — provided a valuable source of information. These nonverbal communications were incredibly beneficial to me as a caregiver.

Likewise, LaVar seemed to look instinctively into my eyes for messages of comfort, encouragement, and reassurance. This alternative form of communication was more accessible than words. Often in medical situations, he looked to me with fear in his eyes because he didn't understand what was happening. With a wink of my eye, he was reassured. I learned to consciously manage my facial expressions — particularly my eyes — so that I could reassure rather than add my distress to his.

Since he no longer drove, LaVar surrendered his driver's license in exchange for a picture identification. Even though I stood by as his photo was taken, I was stunned by the image on the card. His face hung in an expressionless mass; his mouth kind of drooped; it was the face of confusion and distress. Although they looked tired, his eyes were the most familiar feature of his face; they still communicated.

LaVar often commented that an artist's most valuable skill is the ability to see. As a caregiver, I learned to look for LaVar in his eyes where he honestly expressed himself. I learned to see him instead of the outward signs of a disease that was robbing him of life. In LaVar's eyes, I could see the same man that I had known for many years. As difficult as it was, I forced myself to see . . . see how to help . . . see how to comfort . . . see how to love him. LaVar's eyes never stopped communicating until they closed . . . in death.

Music is another effective means of communication and has the power to affect mood. Before Alzheimer's dementia manifested itself, LaVar enjoyed music as a backdrop for his creative work in his studio. He regarded the free form of jazz as the perfect complement to his abstract paintings. When LaVar was agitated, the last thing that I would have incorporated into the situation would have been loud music. Choosing something with a slower tempo and a strong melodic line soothed him. When his mood was upbeat, I could play some old favorite dance music and hold his hands while we sort of danced. Music, like art, is another language and can be used to communicate happiness, peace, and tenderness.

Since I am not an artist, creating a visual message is beyond my comprehension. However, it was through LaVar's final drawings that he created a communication breakthrough with me. It was rather like a Helen Keller/Anne Sullivan experience when I finally understood how deliberately and purposefully he was communicating his emotions, confusion, and distress. After LaVar's death, I realized that what I assumed were subconscious drawings/doodlings were actually profound messages in which he expressed himself. The eyes and faces incorporated into the drawings had the same expressions that I noticed so often in his eyes. I didn't perceive these drawings as communications because I wasn't looking for them. I didn't realize how aware and present an individual with dementia could be. Without a reliable means of assessing what a person suffering with dementia remembers, I see other important considerations. "Is my loved one aware?" "Does he seem glad to see me?" "What can I see in her eyes?" Acting on these higher forms of communication improved my care for LaVar.

A Diagnosis for Two

Don't Straighten
Him Out

Distressing and unpredictable changes in LaVar prompted me to seek additional input. As I expressed my frustrations regarding LaVar's obstinacies, Dr. Helms listened patiently and provided some practical wisdom that guided me through many situations. He simply advised, "Don't try to straighten him out." This became a life-saving piece of advice.

As Alzheimer's dementia progressed, LaVar's unpredictable behavior and volatile reactions made confrontation illogical. It only initiated or escalated conflicts and only served to agitate both of us. Tracking and reintroducing frustrations from earlier moments or even the day before would have created so much unproductive conflict. Therefore, I resisted the urge to seek resolution by talking through disagreements or insisting on an apology. I forced myself to let it go. This tactic was difficult until I realized how much easier it made life for both of us. Then each day presented itself as a new canvas awaiting the brush strokes that would transform it into a work of art.

Letting go of anger or irritation is different than just ignoring it. I tried to use difficult episodes as a signal to play detective. LaVar couldn't help me with this effort, but when I took the time to consider an incident from his point of view, I managed and planned better. For example, I recognized that too much confusion created some processing overload for him. Noisy family gatherings that might have been enjoyable in the past became irritants. One evening as we played games with family, LaVar suddenly retreated to the bedroom. Whenever he heard a cheer, laugh, or other response, he called out in distress. The games had to stop. Because fatigue, pain, or other problems were not things that LaVar could reliably express, it was up to me to understand and advocate for him.

The urge to correct LaVar was more difficult to suppress when we were at a doctor's appointment. Listening to him provide answers to questions and knowing that what he said was untrue, I struggled against the impulse to provide accurate details. Possibly sensing the inaccuracy of LaVar's account, the nurse or doctor glanced at me. At that point, I could offer a discrete shake of my head. It was especially difficult to remain silent when reports made me look irresponsible as a caregiver. My ego wanted to step up to defend, but it wasn't reasonable to use the doctor's time to bicker about differing facts. I just tried to make certain that the specifics were transmitted. I learned that I couldn't "straighten out" someone who has dementia.

A Diagnosis for Two

Not Taking "It" Personally

On another occasion, I burst into tears while recounting frustrations about LaVar's behavior. Dr. Helms offered some additional life-changing advice. Calmly, he said, "Don't take it personally." Later I thought, "It . . . what is an 'it'?" I learned that "it" had many aspects. The first "it" was the disease. LaVar didn't choose to have this affliction. "It" happened to him. Accepting caregiving responsibilities for someone whom I loved was my choice not his. Again, reminding myself that these undesirable changes were not his choice, I could make much better decisions because it was in my control to do so.

"It" caused many challenging personality and behavioral changes. This advice kept me from assuming an ulterior motive for inappropriate behavior and kept me from being angry or resentful. We were out of town visiting family when LaVar suddenly rose to his feet and declared, "I'm out of here." Surprised by this outburst, I tried to calm him and gloss over a shockingly awkward situation. He rejected all of my attempts to restore civility. Recognizing the futility of the situation, I extended an apology, gathered our things, and we left. Certainly, I was embarrassed, frustrated, and yes, even angry, but none of my emotions were ever discussed with LaVar. What would have been accomplished by such debriefing? Driving home, I tried to keep some happy chatter going to lighten his mood. When he continued to brood, I stopped to get his favorite fast-food meal, which seemed to help. I never tracked down a reasonable cause of the incident, but I didn't take "it" personally.

Memories of shared experiences are precious. Although I believe that it's impossible to assess a dementia patient's recall adequately, it can be difficult not to take "it" personally when a loved one can't retrieve a tender moment. For at least a year and a half before he died, LaVar did not know my name. I became suspicious when he stopped calling our dogs by their names and for a time called them "dogs" and then progressed to "things." As we traveled in the car, I queried, "Do you know my name?" LaVar neither hesitated nor seem disturbed as he replied, "Nope." I pressed with, "Do you know who I am?" He brightened declaring, "Yes, you're the lady who does stuff for us." Indeed! We went to get ice cream. His reply told me that although he couldn't provide my name, he trusted me and relied on my kindness. He didn't need to recall my name because I knew it the whole time. I didn't take "it" personally when he couldn't remember something.

A Diagnosis for Two

Less Is More

More is an interesting word—more accomplishments, more entertainment, more things, more vacations. I learned to appreciate the power of less. Yes, I own a planner and filled it with numerous tasks each day during my career. However, in caring for LaVar, I learned that having an absolute deadline was a disaster in waiting. Efficiency became a sworn enemy of effectiveness. My power as a caregiver was to set the pace of the day according to circumstances and adapt as needed. That flexibility could be awkward when plans involved others.

Productivity was something that LaVar prized highly. Prior to the onset of Alzheimer's dementia, he was a prolific artist and went to his studio with clear objectives. He looked forward to waking in the morning and often waited impatiently for me to leave for my office so that he could get to work. He created in a wide variety of mediums and often produced a series of items. Sometimes his studio was filled with watercolor paintings, and other times pottery covered the tables. He was productive and relished showing me his accomplishments when I came home from work.

Retiring to become LaVar's caregiver, I assumed that he would be drawn to his studio and reengage the many art projects that had occupied him previously. Instead, he wanted to sleep in, shave and shower, and eat a tasty breakfast. If I had tried to impose a schedule with prioritized tasks on it, every day would have been a disaster. On the days when we had appointments or other activities that required conforming to a schedule, the day was neither as peaceful nor, ultimately, as productive.

Slowing down was extremely hard for me, but it was one of the best things that I did as a caregiver. Once I begin a project, I like to finish. A specific example comes to mind. I was taking pieces of art from high display areas so that I could clean them. LaVar helped by taking the items out of my hands. Without warning he sat down on the sofa while still holding a small sculpture. He seemed perturbed as though something unpleasant had just happened. In analyzing the situation, I realized that he was probably confused by what I was doing with "his stuff," and perhaps he was becoming tired. Sensing the change in his mood, I put away the ladder, pushed everything aside, and suggested that we go for a drive to get some ice cream.

Afterward, we sat on the couch while he dozed. It took much longer to finish the project than I had planned, but the adjustment yielded a far better outcome.

LaVar loved to garden and to do yard work. As dementia progressed, I had to manage the size and scope of work projects since his energy levels lagged. The last time that he planted a garden, we took turns running the rototiller. Finishing a mowing project in one day wasn't always possible. Sometimes I had to finish up after LaVar went to bed or even the next day. Again, not in keeping with my personal style or preference, but it was the smart thing to do.

A Diagnosis for Two

The Power of Distraction

Often older adults express frustration about losing their train of thought, the inability to find the right word, or misplacing something. Loss of attention is susceptible to even slight distractions. For most, this lapse is an annoyance. However, in some situations a distraction can be disastrous — driving for example. As a teacher, I monitored the students' focus in order to make adaptations as needed. "Pay attention," was a common reminder. However, I learned that distraction was a powerful tool for me as a caregiver. Using diversions strategically allowed me to deflect LaVar's focus and curb a pending incident.

Routines can be comforting as long as the schedule doesn't override flexibility. Each day I tried to quickly assess LaVar's mood and adapt accordingly. One morning LaVar slept later than usual and awoke after I had left the bedroom. In an attempt to take care of himself, he began putting on clothes. His robe was on one shoulder with his light jacket on the other arm. He put on all of his wrist watches. He put on his pants and shoes; clearly, he was getting ready for something. Rather than trying to back up for the normal morning procedure of shave, shower, and dress, I suggested that we have some super delicious breakfast. With a cheery lilt in my voice, I chatted with him while he ate some favorite breakfast foods. This distraction interrupted the dressing that was becoming increasingly frustrating and offered him something soothing instead. After eating, it was easy to get LaVar back into the bathroom for bathing and dressing. Later I wondered whether the underlying issue was hunger; I couldn't be sure; it didn't matter. Without the ability to express himself, I had to use my judgment to make the best decision. I wasn't always right. Respecting his individuality and preferences ahead of my own agenda or routine was an incredibly useful strategy. Distracting LaVar with his favorite things worked 100 percent of the time.

Many caregivers struggle with the aggravation of repeated questions. Perhaps these inquiries are an expression of confusion or even anxiety. Distraction was a handy strategy for this problem, too. I tried to keep things around that engaged LaVar's hands. Since he liked to create in a variety of mediums. A small box of magnetic toys was a ready distraction. He also liked greeting cards, so a stack of cards that

I had given him for various occasions was useful. A magazine or newspaper could provide a few minutes of distraction as well. Until he lost the ability to talk without frustration, I could distract LaVar with my own questions. "Where would you like to go for a drive?" "What would you like to have for dinner?" "What is the weather like?" Even if his responses didn't make sense, I let him talk. When LaVar became involved in expressing something, the repeated questions stopped. Even just talking to him was soothing especially if my tone of voice was calm and cheerful.

Projects are great distractors and a favorite activity can derail an outburst. Some like puzzles . . . using the hands can be a great way to calm the mind. On one occasion, I impulsively pulled the silverware tray out of the drawer, dumped it onto the kitchen island, and asked LaVar to help me put it back together. Sorting provided an effective interruption. Sensing that fatigue could be the problem, I distracted LaVar with a warm blanket and a hand rub that brought on a little nap. Sleep usually restored a better mood.

Sometimes I had to use a series of distractions to interrupt an unpleasant episode. LaVar was at work with me as my staff and I prepared a light snack for an upcoming staff meeting. Observing as we arranged the food, LaVar took a small cluster of grapes. One of my staff commented in a teasing tone, "Are you sneaking some food?" He returned immediately to my office in foul humor. When I couldn't coax him out of his bad mood, I suggested that we take a drive and took him home. Even being in a familiar environment didn't calm him, so I provided another distraction.

A blue spruce shrub had outgrown its space in our landscaping and needed some trimming. We went outside and began working together. Noticing that LaVar was using his little clipper to cut branches that I intended to keep, I wanted to stop him but resisted saying anything. The shrub was ruined; the day was saved. A negative reaction from me could have ignited another incident. Instead, I let my secretary know that I wouldn't be attending the meeting, offered LaVar a sandwich and a cup of soup, and chatted happily about our wonderful work. His mood was good; it was a pleasant evening; he slept well. All of those positive outcomes were due to the effective use of distraction. At a later time, some friends came to visit and cut down the shrub. I incorporated its skeleton into the landscape of our yard as a ready reminder that being flexible is always the best approach when dealing with a human being who doesn't understand. It's a tangible type of kindness. Avoiding outbursts is the most powerful way of coping with them.

Indeed, caregiving had numerous lessons to offer. As soon as I found a way to navigate around a problem, another situation appeared that required yet another unique answer. Flexibility in caring for another helped me to be nimble and resilient. During a time of chronic change and intense learning, I came to appreciate the power of kindness in soothing someone suffering with dementia. Kindness was my most reliable ally.

A Diagnosis for Two

The Decline

Seemingly out of nowhere, green summer landscape is replaced by the drying, yellowing vegetation of fall; no human effort stops nature's transition. Likewise, LaVar's declining health was a time to accept changes and generate as much happiness as possible. Many previously enjoyable diversions became "last time" occasions as LaVar experienced a succession of declines.

"What's the matter with me? I barely even know who I am." LaVar blurted out unexpectedly. Only moments before, he had been peacefully napping on the living room couch. His clarity of thought and his ability to express himself was shocking because his verbal language was almost nonexistent. Searching for a way to explain the inexplicable, I delayed my response by putting away the folded laundry. Composing myself before looking into his eyes, I offered, "You have been diagnosed with Alzheimer's dementia." We cried together; he understood. In a few minutes, LaVar stated rather matter of factly, "I have to get out of here. I can't stand to go through what my mother did." I asked him what he wanted me to do, and he offered some guidance. The flash of clarity was gone almost as quickly as it appeared. From that moment, his decline was precipitous. Every day brought new challenges or difficulties.

At first the problem of incontinence was an occasional nuisance, a minor inconvenience, that I addressed by trying to be vigilant about regular bathroom breaks. Soon the problem created mountains of laundry. Instead of addressing incontinence matter-of-factly, I just washed bedding and many changes of clothes each day. I was concerned that broaching the issue of adult protection products would upset LaVar and set off an unpleasant episode. However, one day as I helped him change, he said, "That damn dog peed my pants." It was such a charming expression of innocence that I giggled. Seeing my response, he laughed, too. Then I suggested that we go to the store to pick out some stuff that would help with the problem. It was so much easier than I had imagined. It was not a problem that LaVar could control, and I couldn't resolve it with complaints or dialogue. Once this problem appeared, it never ended; it was a milepost of decline. No amount of extra work on my part could fix it.

Coming home after a long, busy day, we entered our home after dark. We hardly came into the back

hallway when LaVar began yelling, "Give me my keys!"
When I tried to explain that I didn't have them, his
agitation escalated, and he began throwing things. It
was the first time that I feared for my safety. Although
I wanted to flee, I was afraid to leave him alone. My
son responded to my distress call and parked on the
driveway in case he needed to intervene. He coached
me by phone regarding possible measures to calm
LaVar. Following the recommendations, I was able to
get him to fall asleep in a comfortable chair.

Gently rousing him later, I told him that he had fallen
asleep, and now it was time to go to bed. Tenderly,
I tucked him in, and he slept soundly. The next
morning, LaVar noticed a couple of broken items;
I dismissed them nonchalantly. No part of that
terrible, frightening night came forward — it was
forgotten — erased. In spite of the unpredictability of
Alzheimer's dementia, each day represented a blank
slate. The challenging part for me was to forget as
well. However, that incident was a sobering reminder
that things were changing, and I needed to develop
additional strategies.

Caregiving became increasingly unpredictable. LaVar
had nightmares that made him call out in his sleep and
flail his arms as though he were fighting off something
dangerous. He sometimes fell out of bed due to a
night fright. With the loss of verbal communication,
he couldn't articulate the cause; I just tried to soothe

him so that he could go back to sleep. Other times LaVar was able to express the source of his distress. One night he awoke sobbing because a loved one never came to see him. It was an accurate statement but nothing that I could control.

Daily, I struggled to incorporate enjoyable activities that had previously filled hours — a search for something that felt "normal." I was reluctant to accept that things were deteriorating in spite of my heroic efforts. It was in experiencing the frustration and futility of my best attempts that I realized that some activities were no longer possible. As LaVar and I shopped in a large store, he pushed the shopping cart while I gathered our purchases. It provided some exercise and a diversion from our home routine. As we left the store that day, he declared, "No more!" It was pointless to insist or to inquire about the reasons. It was our last shopping trip there.

Dining out became impossible when it presented a safety issue. While eating at a favorite restaurant with some friends, LaVar stood up and walked outside without warning. Since the business was located on a busy street, I followed to make certain that he didn't wander into traffic. After roaming around the parking lot for a few minutes, he went to our car and got inside. I remarked that I had forgotten something and would be right back. I paid the check, offered apologies to our friends, and drove LaVar home. It was the last time to dine out.

The Decline

We enjoyed soaking in private pools at a nearby hot springs. Knowing how much LaVar appreciated the soothing water's effects on sore joints and muscles, I took him regularly. This time he became sullen and refused to change into his swimming suit. Thinking that he might be confused, I changed into my suit. When he still resisted, I got into the pool and tried to entice him with a description of how wonderful the water felt. He became even more aggravated. Realizing that the situation was not going to improve, I got out, dressed, and drove home. It was a last soak.

LaVar loved to bowl and participated on a league when he was a young adult. Now he mostly sat at the scoring table and observed. The last time that we went bowling, the grandchildren urged him to join in. Unexpectedly accepting the challenge, he held up the bowling ball and looked over his shoulder with such a joyful smile. Although it's impossible to know what sparked that involvement, we were charmed by his obvious enjoyment. His was the highest score on this last game. It was his last strike.

Whenever someone asked LaVar to explain a work of art, he remarked that he often worked out of his subconscious when creating. Reasoning that he might function better in his art studio than anywhere else, I accompanied him and worked at my makeshift desk. Since he referred to pottery as "his touchstone medium," I suggested that he throw some pots. My assistance was not much help since I'm not an artist, but once LaVar sat at the wheel, pots appeared. Soon a table was covered with various shapes and sizes of drying vessels. I was elated to see something that resembled "normal" for LaVar. He trimmed the pots and carved some of them before returning them to the table to dry thoroughly before the first firing.

LaVar's stamina was lagging, so a morning's work was usually the extent of his effort. It was only a glimpse of a former time, but the hope of normalcy faded with each phase of production. In an episode of agitation, LaVar smashed many of the drying pots. It was like watching him play "Whack a Mole." Although I was distressed by the destruction, nothing could have stopped him. Later the surviving pots advanced to their first firing. Again my own inexperience and lack of knowledge wasn't helpful. I thought that the way that LaVar loaded the kiln was odd but didn't intervene. Alas, when the firing was completed, many pots were broken. The remaining pieces advanced to the decorating and glazing phase. Again, this effort revealed that LaVar had lost control of the processes and materials. When he tried to decorate a pot with some acrylic paint, without thinking, I blurted out, "No, that's not right." He shot me a look of defiance and continued. When the kiln door opened on the last firing, LaVar reached in and handed me a beautifully carved flat plate. The glorious colors and interesting glazes that once blazed in the sunlight now were a dull brown when the door opened. LaVar's ability to mix and apply the glaze was gone. It was a disappointing outcome — LaVar's last pottery project.

LaVar loved to make jewelry for me, and as a special occasion approached, I asked him if he wanted to go to his studio. Indeed, the results of his efforts were not his finest work, but it was wonderful to watch him diligently and lovingly create. The evidence of brain disease was obvious as he struggled with the materials and tools. When he became frustrated, I tried to help, but he seemed annoyed by my intervention. My only option was to monitor his safety and let him do whatever he wanted. It was the last time that he produced jewelry.

LaVar worked diligently on a highly textured acrylic painting. The scene emerged in glorious colors with amazing strata. Later I glanced over as LaVar covered the entire canvas with white paint in wide, purposeful strokes. Distressed to see the nearly completed painting ruined, I blurted out, "Why did you do that?" LaVar looked at me with a blank expression and completely ignored my question. After letting the paint dry, he began painting the same scene, but again, the nearly completed landscape received a white coating. It was difficult to watch this process repeat itself, but expecting the "old normal" would have created so much more distress for LaVar and for me. Instead, I bought a ridiculous amount of white paint and let go. LaVar's paintings were complete; his lifetime of art was drawing to a close.

Knowing how much LaVar enjoyed going to the Oregon coast, we accepted an invitation to join my son's family for a few days at an ocean-side resort. Preparing for the trip was challenging. Sensing that something out of the ordinary was happening, LaVar became agitated and unpleasant. I immediately stopped the preparations until he fell asleep for the night. The next morning, I helped him clean up as usual and fed him breakfast. Then I helped him into the car, and we were on our way. In retrospect, it was probably dangerous to be in the car for long distances, but I was searching desperately for ways to engage him in activities that he enjoyed. I yearned for our old life.

LaVar and I loved the ocean and delighted in its sights and sounds. We took every opportunity to walk on the beach where he looked for interesting rocks and seashells. All of us in our group stayed close by him even though his pace was unusually slow. As we prepared to return to the car, LaVar fell to his hands and knees. He had a walking stick, but he couldn't use it to help himself. We all lifted and helped him back to the car. Wistfully, I stood watching as the tide went out for our last time.

Searching for the perfect present as LaVar's last birthday approached, I decided to give him an experience as his gift. Together we bought the ingredients for his favorite meal: pot roast, potatoes, carrots, and his amazing chocolate cake. He looked so natural and seemed incredibly happy as he peeled vegetables while the pot roast seared in a pan that he had used for many years. The cake batter swallowed the chocolate chips and walnuts. While the cake baked, we prepared the butter cream frosting. When the creation was assembled, LaVar sprinkled miniature chocolate chips on top. It was a masterpiece . . . it was an accomplishment . . . it was an expression of love. As he sat at the table, his face radiated a look of joy. It may have been the best gift that I ever gave him; it was an acknowledgment of his individuality, preferences, and abilities. It was the last supper that he ever made.

LaVar and I loved to travel and spent many happy hours appreciating the beautiful and varied scenery while traveling to various destinations. As we drove through central Idaho on our way to Coeur d'Alene, we admired the velvety green mountain slopes. The overcast skies lent a misty quality to the scene where evidence of snow clung to highland slopes. LaVar intently studied those awe-inspiring vistas. Nevertheless, my hope for a perfect day was short lived. In spite of my best preparations for a serene day, about 100 miles from our destination, LaVar demanded, "Take me home!" I reassured him that we would be going home soon and kept driving. Rest stops were difficult because increasingly he needed help at facilities not suited for caregiver assistance. His agitation grew, and my fear increased as we traveled the last miles.

When we arrived at our destination, our family welcomed LaVar with a special dinner treat of hot rolls, chicken thighs, and mashed potatoes. It was a perfect diversion. After eating he sat at the table as we talked until quite late and seemed to enjoy the evening. The next day, we went to see the farm progress. Although the terrain was sticky, slick-clay mud, LaVar trudged along looking at and petting the animals. On our return to the vehicles, LaVar slumped to the ground and couldn't continue. All of us helped him to his feet and back into the car. It was his last farm visit.

Later that morning, LaVar and I drove to the Tri-cities in Washington where we spent a few days with my brother. This part of the trip was easier because it was a shorter distance. LaVar settled in on the family room couch and listened to the chatter. During our visit, he ate and slept well; it was remarkably pleasant. One afternoon a pile of junk mail on the kitchen island attracted LaVar's attention. He pulled up a stool and began opening and sorting the letters. It's impossible to know what he was thinking.

When the weather offered a sunny, warm afternoon, we bought food and headed to the river park for a picnic. After eating LaVar tossed chunks of bread to the ducks and geese. He looked over his shoulder and flashed a joyous look—pure happiness. On our final day there, we ran several errands. With each stop, it became more difficult for LaVar to get in and out of the car. His increasing frailty was evident; stepping over a curb in a parking lot was difficult and risky. When we stopped for ice cream, LaVar wouldn't get out of the car but remarked, "The lady will bring me some." For sure she did—his favorite kind.

As I helped him change for bed that night, he said, "I had the nicest day with your mother." Since I was the only woman present, I asked, "Do you mean me?" He said adamantly, "No, it was your mother!" My mother had been dead for more than 45 years. The next morning, we returned to our home. These traveling adventures forced me to see that it was not reasonable anymore—it was our final vacation.

Since LaVar loved people, I tried to arrange visits whenever he brought up someone's name repeatedly. If he couldn't get out of the car and go inside, friends came to the car to visit with him. Nevertheless, he always seemed happy to see his friends and former colleagues. When he kept mentioning a weaving student from his early years of teaching, I located her. Now well into her 90's, she lived in her own home with her daughter's assistance. Delighted to see her mentor and long-time friend, this lady welcomed us and showed LaVar items that she had woven recently as well as projects still on the loom. He seemed interested but didn't say anything. After we sat down in the living room, the lady looked at him quizzically. Clearly, she realized that something was wrong. Since I never discussed LaVar's condition in front of him, the topic was not addressed. It was a last visit.

LaVar loved his sister and had begun saying her name often even in the middle of the night. I arranged a meeting and drove 300 miles so that he could see her. As we walked into a busy, noisy restaurant for a lunch gathering, LaVar saw his sister from a distance and called out to her by name. It was shocking to me that he could recognize her and come up with her name even in that chaotic environment. We sat together at a table, but he wouldn't eat. When I drove to our hotel later, LaVar demanded, "Take me home." Although it was already evening, he was resolute, so I drove home. After that day, he didn't mention his sister again. It was a final family reunion.

In spite of my best efforts to engage LaVar in activities that were personally enjoyable for him, caregiving became increasingly unpredictable when he began suffering with sundowner's syndrome. As afternoon sun gave way to twilight, LaVar became restless and increasingly agitated. I tried getting him to bed before darkness could upset him, but daily, it became more challenging. LaVar's safety became a greater concern when he left our bedroom quietly one night. Fortunately, our dog awakened me before LaVar got too far away from the door. Now my sleep was no longer restful because I knew that the danger of his wandering was real.

The most serious incident occurred when visitors overstayed and delayed my getting LaVar into bed at a reasonable time. Repeatedly, I went to his side of the bed and tucked him in, but before I could get into bed myself, he was standing by the side of the bed. When he finally fell asleep, I drifted into a restless slumber of exhaustion. Sometime during the early morning hours, I heard a crash. He had fallen against the dresser in our bedroom and scraped his back. Certainly, he was confused and disoriented. When I reached out to help him up, he began swinging at me as though fighting off an attacker. Knowing that I couldn't help him while he was so agitated, I covered him with a warm blanket and turned off the lights. After a short time, I helped him up and back into bed. The next day he was moody and volatile. It was the final alert that my solo caregiving was no longer adequate. LaVar was a large person, so I could neither restrain him from doing something potentially dangerous to himself nor to me.

In consulting with LaVar's doctor, I had to accept that the time had come to get other help since one person cannot provide 24/7 care for another. My first job as a caregiver was to keep LaVar safe, and if I could no longer insure that, my choices were limited. Respite care was not working because he didn't understand why another person was in our home. He relied solely on me to take care of him. Although letting go seems to suggest surrender, for me it was a recognition that circumstances were beyond my control. This was easily the most difficult phase of caregiving because I was forced to acknowledge that I had hit my limit. Events in the last few months of his life presented hurdles that I could neither ignore nor surmount. When considering safety, the decision was apparent.

Months before LaVar and I visited several facilities in order to explore options. I had considered going to an assisted-living facility with him in order to get some help and still be together. Now I could see that the facility best for him was a small group home where all of the residents had a dementia diagnosis. Gathering LaVar's things was difficult for me because I knew how distressing this change would be for both of us. The only thing that kept me moving forward was knowing and really accepting that I couldn't offer enough care.

Some family came to help me with the transition. We shared LaVar's favorite breakfast and lunch; then it was time to go. He looked suspiciously at the baskets of clothing loaded into the cars. When we got to the facility, we all went in, so he followed. When he saw me unpacking clothing into the dresser drawers, he became agitated. Several individuals tried to distract him while I filled out the necessary paperwork. I opted for respite care rather than permanent placement because I was too conflicted about leaving him. At one point, LaVar burst into the office with a horrible look of confusion and anger on his face. Clearly, he knew that something was happening.

Witnessing that exchange, the administrator suggested that I not come back for three to five days so that LaVar could adjust. In that amount of time, she reassured, he would forget about me and accept the staff and other residents as his new family. Then I could be his wife instead of his caregiver. That suggestion, even now, remains with me as evidence of how dehumanizing Alzheimer's disease and other dementing illnesses are. Even if LaVar could forget about me, my options weren't so clear. Heartbroken, I drew comfort from knowing that I had done everything that I could.

After one miserable day, I realized that I couldn't bear to be away from LaVar. Entering the facility, I saw him looking confused and distressed. With a cheerful greeting, I asked if he would like to clean up. He cooperated as I helped him shave, shower, and dress. Then the staff made a special hot breakfast for him. Everyone was so amazed at his mood change. Roaming the hallways constantly, he had become a fearful presence. Each day thereafter I spent long hours at the facility with LaVar in order to comfort him and to help him adapt. Daily I showered and dressed him. Several professionals suggested that providing LaVar with daily showers was too much because the state standard was twice a week. When setting criteria for an anonymous group of people, it is easier to set that standard. However, respecting LaVar's individual preference, I offered him the daily care that pleased him. Desperately, I searched for other alternatives, but I couldn't devise a plan for caregiving that didn't include sleep. Also, agitation can lead to aggression, and it was my responsibility to insure everyone's safety, including my own. LaVar would not have wanted to hurt me; he didn't. Knowing that I had already contributed everything that I could brought peace. Then letting go became an act of love.

Burdened by knowing how unhappy LaVar was, I impulsively went to the facility one morning and brought him home. He was so happy. Our dogs greeted him joyfully as he entered the house; he ignored them. I made him some breakfast; he ate only a couple of bites. He toured through the house and closely examined all of his paintings, pottery, and sculpture. It was as though he were visiting a museum and admiring the beautiful art work. Then he sat on the couch and fell asleep. While he rested, I prepared some more of his favorite foods; again, he wouldn't eat. When I raised a forkful of food to his lips, he gruffly said, "Don't!"

As the afternoon gave way to evening, LaVar began
to get restless. He opened the back door and headed
out to the deck. Knowing that he would not be able
to navigate the stairs, I tried to redirect him. He
became agitated by my efforts; I was frightened. No
one knew that I had taken him home, and I could see
that we were both in danger. Coaxing him into the
car, I drove back to the facility. Once there I helped
him inside where he immediately disappeared into
another resident's room. That day reaffirmed that I
could not manage LaVar at home any longer. It was
a beautiful but devastating day—a confirmation that I
had indeed done all that I could.

The final evening of LaVar's life was a culmination
of a difficult day. His visual perception was so
compromised that he couldn't judge the transition
between tile and carpet on the floors. The staff
brought a walker to help steady him, but it was too
complicated. He couldn't manage to sit down in a
wheelchair. Finally, I pulled him to the edge of the
bed to sit beside me. Holding hands, our fingers
laced together. The strong hands that had served,
created, and protected were now in need of care.
"Please, God, don't make us suffer more than we can
bear," I offered aloud. LaVar struggled to his feet
in a few minutes and then began falling backwards.
Fortunately, I was able to stop his fall. The staff put
him into bed, and I went home. The next morning,

preparing to shower and dress, I received a phone call that LaVar was gone . . . "Where did he go?" I asked. He was really gone — time to rest.

Caregiver Reflection

As I write, winter approaches; days shorten; light dims. Mounds of newly fallen snow shroud the landscape. Sitting in stillness, I reflect upon the transformative lessons of caregiving. Indeed, my experiences with Alzheimer's dementia enlightened me in unanticipated ways and changed me in ways that I cherish. The memories have become beautiful. Even suggesting that there is anything attractive about such a difficult and tragic disease is a bold statement since the word beauty suggests something appealing. Certainly, Alzheimer's dementia or any other dementing illness wouldn't immediately bring pleasant associations to mind. Possibly, the things that I cherish most were not incidental to the disease itself but to personal adaptations that circumstances forced upon me. Ideally, I try to live life forward because ruminating on the past wastes energy on things that cannot be changed and leads to regret. However, reflection is a phase of learning in which experiences become more integrated and useful in other situations. In part this reflection on my caregiving experience is intended to help others who currently care for someone.

Seeing the first signs of odd behaviors, I didn't seek a diagnosis. Perhaps it was my assumption that nothing could be done even if it were Alzheimer's dementia. Additionally, since LaVar was approaching 80, I didn't have enough experience to distinguish between disease and normal aging. Today I would pursue a diagnosis in order to have clarity that helps any caregiver make better choices. Nearly 10 years have passed since I struggled with those first signs, and although pharmaceutical options are still lacking, lifestyle recommendations, though challenging to implement, would have guided me. Honestly, I used food and activities to comfort LaVar rather than treat his condition. With an early diagnosis, I would have had better medical guidance instead of operating on my instincts. Early intervention is still the best possible approach.

Interacting with LaVar as he suffered with Alzheimer's dementia was enlightening, but other acquaintances with dementia have reinforced my insights. The most profound lesson that I learned about dementia was how aware individuals are even though they can't communicate as they did in the past. Sounds and motions replace words; behaviors replace other expressions of need. Memories are not gone although retrieval isn't reliable. I muse about the many observations that LaVar blurted out with shocking clarity and accuracy; it was counter to everything that I had read or had been told. Until he had a communication breakthrough with me near the end of his life and spent his last days thereafter creating messages, I viewed these occasions with curiosity. Now I know better.

Caregiving is a difficult role to fulfill alone; all caregivers need help. It was hard for me to ask for assistance because I didn't understand what was needed. Every day was filled with new challenges for which I had neither a plan nor prior experience. When struggling with life's other difficulties, I assumed that circumstances would improve with time. However, with Alzheimer's dementia each day became harder, more difficult, more challenging, more exhausting. Offers for help were mostly nonexistent because the house was clean, meals were prepared, and the yard looked as lovely as ever. No one perceived the amount of struggle involved in maintaining our lifestyle. In reflecting on the situation, I should have reached out for help because others would have responded. Difficult days should have prompted me to identify options and gather resources. A challenging present is a call to action. No one else can recognize another's tipping point.

Isolation is a difficult aspect of dementia for the
patient as well as the caregiver. Rationally, I
understand that seeing a loved one decline and lose
many of the traits that once defined a relationship is
tough. Possibly operating on the assumption that a
loved one won't remember anyway makes it seem less
important. As LaVar declined, we spent most of our
days alone. When an infrequent visitor came, LaVar
seemed happy, and even though he couldn't contribute
to the conversation, he leaned forward as though
ready to say something. Speaking is different than
listening; remembering is different than being aware.

LaVar and I were fortunate because we enjoyed being
together; otherwise, the constancy of our togetherness
would have been a frustration. I recognize that not
all relationships are like that, and it's okay. However,
I believe that the presence of a caring human being is
important for anyone who is experiencing confusion
and distress. Does that human need change that much
over the course of a lifetime? It seems to me that the
need for kindness is fairly constant.

Watching a talented and productive human reduced
to a man who needed constant care and supervision
was difficult. However, I wonder how frustrating it
must have been for LaVar to have someone monitor,
mediate, and correct his efforts to perform previously
routine tasks. Having to offer assistance with
personal care can be difficult and even unpleasant

for a caregiver, but I can't imagine the indignities of receiving that kind of help. Witnessing my struggles and stress as LaVar declined, some offered the glib advice, "Just put him somewhere and go on with your life." Perhaps it's reasonable to assume that placing a loved one in the care of others would be a relief rather than a grief.

I suppose that everyone has worst-case dreads—fears that one hopes to never encounter. For me it is a dementing illness because of how I observed it strip away individuality, dignity, and independence. Creating generalizations about a group of humans who cannot speak for themselves leads to treating those who have a similar illness as though they share identical characteristics and needs. It was horrifying to witness how Alzheimer's dementia seemed to replace LaVar's identity. If he had cancer, his wishes would have been respected. If he had been comatose, loved ones would have been encouraged to interact with him. As soon as memory faded and the ability to communicate was compromised, it was easy for others to assume that he was "gone."

LaVar's life with Alzheimer's dementia would have been much different if I had believed that he was no longer the individual whom I knew. My approach to caregiving was based upon knowing his preferences and offering them to him. For example, although he loved to cook, increasingly the processes became too difficult. However, I facilitated his participation by allowing him to work alongside me. The particular task didn't seem to matter; being involved provided obvious enjoyment.

Beyond honoring the individuality of those with dementia, identifying preferences provides direction for caregivers. A plan to offer enjoyable entertainment or participation in hobbies and leisure activities acknowledges that preferences are still intact. Not all music is soothing to everyone. Food preferences still exist, and social inclinations are still there. A human with dementia is still an individual. The downside of my caregiving approach was that it was difficult for me to accept that it was time to just settle in and create a tranquil environment. In reflecting on LaVar's final descent, I know that his energy and strength were failing, and he lacked the stamina to enjoy some activities that I provided for him.

In reflection I remember how caring for a vulnerable adult with a degenerative brain disease is notably different than any other type of caregiving. I could neither teach nor train LaVar to follow correct procedures; it was pointless to scold him for not following the "rules." Increasingly, his behaviors became illogical and even dangerous. It was as though LaVar declined in reverse to an infant/child's growth and development. Although it occurred unpredictably, independence was steadily replaced by dependence.

Rather than celebrate accomplishments, I had to adapt and to accept. Alzheimer's dementia stripped away the reason and predictability of an adult relationship, so deciding to be flexible became a beautiful gift. Being rigid and demanding as a caregiver would have turned my life into a battleground, and I would have lost the war.

The complex role of caregiving does not generate profuse gratitude. As Alzheimer's dementia progressed, the normally polite and kind LaVar no longer said "please" or "thank you." He seemed oblivious to my stress and fatigue. I'm certain that he didn't grasp my efforts to take care of everything. However, I expected neither accolades nor notes of appreciation. It was an offering—my choice. Keeping in mind that I had accepted a difficult role kept me from venting my frustrations in LaVar's presence. Hearing caregivers share raw, personal details of their experiences makes me cringe as I look to the one with dementia who "doesn't know." Although it's difficult to assess what is being processed and remembered, I learned that the ability to upload emotion is rather profound. Cataloging and rehearsing moments of confusion and distress allows negative experiences to compound and make every day a torture. I resisted getting caught up in senseless conflicts and petty complaints even though there were plenty of opportunities. I tried to appreciate the beauty of offering LaVar compassion.

A Diagnosis for Two

One of the most difficult aspects of caregiving was trying to take care of myself in addition to LaVar. I tried to follow healthful practices and to include exercise because if my health failed, it would have been a disaster for both of us. Even though my efforts were not perfect, I learned to appreciate that physical exercise was a release for my emotions. I felt renewed even though the time to exercise often required a sacrifice of early-morning sleep. Taking care of myself was one aspect of my caregiving role that did not end with LaVar's death.

Simplicity has many gifts to offer and lessons to teach. It provides clarity about what is really important and what is only nice. Maintaining life as I once knew it was impossible; no amount of desperate struggle would have made it better. Rather, it was in celebrating minor accomplishments and appreciating small things that treasured moments came into my life as a caregiver. I learned to live life one day at a time and appreciate the gift of a fresh 24 hours. I learned the beauty of forgetting. The most deeply satisfying aspect of caregiving is the realization that I was able to give hands and feet to my love for LaVar by extending the compassion that he needed and deserved. Whenever I have felt the sting of grief at his death, it has been tempered with the knowledge that I gave him the most beautiful gift that one human being can offer another—kindness.